WE'VE ALL FELT THAT DEFEAT: thumbing through blouse after blouse in your closet, feeling like you have absolutely nothing to wear. Or at least, nothing you feel good in. That's where *Style for Everybody* comes in. Stylist Kim Appelt delivers your go-to fashion road map, sharing the secrets to building a capsule wardrobe for all body shapes and personal styles.

Style for Everybody is filled with fun, approachable style wisdom, including how to:

- ✦ Determine your body shape and personal style
- ✦ Build a new, curated wardrobe, focusing on key garments, shoes, purses, and accessories for each body type and style
- ✦ Condense your current closet with sustainable donation suggestions
- ✦ Shop with efficiency and purpose

With an understanding of versatile body shapes (hourglass and rectangle are only the beginning) and fashion styles (a little preppy, full-on edgy?), Kim recognizes that the better you feel about yourself, the more of a positive force you can be in the world. Filled with inclusive and supportive fashion advice, easy-to-follow style charts for each body shape, and beautiful illustrations, *Style for Everybody* is like having a personal stylist (and cheerleader!) in your home—its encouraging guidance will keep you coming back whenever you need a style pick-

Style for Everybody

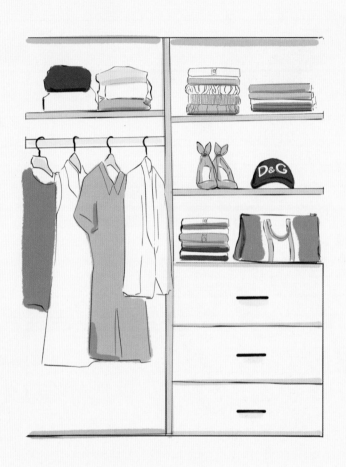

Style for

Everybody

A Guide to Curating
Your Essential Wardrobe

KIM APPELT

appetite

Appetite by Random House® and colophon are registered trademarks of Penguin Random House LLC.

Library and Archives Canada Cataloguing in Publication is available upon request.

ISBN: 9780525612216
eBook ISBN: 9780525612223

Book design: Kate Sinclair
Interior illustrations: Nessa Wiktorczyk

Printed in China

Published in Canada by Appetite by Random House®,
a division of Penguin Random House Canada Limited.

www.penguinrandomhouse.ca

10 9 8 7 6 5 4 3 2 1

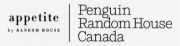

appetite
by RANDOM HOUSE

Penguin
Random House
Canada

Gratitude to the One that has always
walked ahead of me and opened the doors.

cont

Introduction   1

1. Getting Started   9

2. The Dragon's Lair   25

3. Putting It All Together   41

4. The It List   49

5. Essential Footwear   63

ents

6. Essential Purses   75

7. Essential Accessories   87

8. How to Shop   103

9. How to Actually Get Dressed   117

Style Charts   129

Acknowledgments   153

Introduction

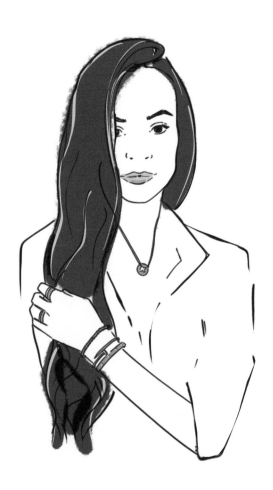

For as long as I can remember, I have been dressing people. My early years were spent growing up in Gaborone, Botswana. I'm unsure if it was my mom and dad's parenting style or the slow arrival of our treasured belongings, but for a while my siblings and I didn't have as many toys as we had had in North America. As a result of our low supply of playthings, we had to get more creative, and I took to styling at an early age as a form of entertainment. My first and very willing participant was my little sister, Kristin. Four years my junior, Kristin didn't seem to mind being dressed and undressed repeatedly. I would create "wigs" out of my mother's nylons and stunning "frocks" from kitchen aprons, and once these delightful creations were finished, I would dress her up and place a wig on her small head to create a long princess-like braid. She never objected. The smile on

Being with my
mom when she
looked and
felt great was
contagious—it
made me feel
great, too!

her face as she got in her chariot (aka the wheelbarrow) made my heart beat faster. It was at that early age that my desire to style was cemented.

We returned to North America five years later, and I remember watching my mom as she took care getting dressed and putting on makeup—even just for a trip to the grocery store. I once asked her why she bothered to look good just to run errands. Her eyes twinkled as she replied, "The question, Kimberley, is why wouldn't you? It's fun, and I feel good." That was enough for me. It confirmed the happiness that can be derived from looking and feeling great. And being with my mom when she looked and felt great was contagious—it made me feel great, too!

As I grew up, my fascination with styling continued. I dressed my best friend, Paula, for our grade 6 dance. Neither of us had any new clothes, so she borrowed a few pieces from another friend and I put together our looks. I started modelling at 16, and being the budding stylist that I was, I couldn't resist helping to pull the looks together on set and dress the other models. The other girls were more timid than I was, and I made them laugh and feel good about themselves, which always made for a better shoot. In my university days, my friends would come over to my place, knowing they could arrive wearing whatever and there would be a dramatic overhaul before we hit the town. I intuitively understood body shape and dressing according to personal style but wasn't yet able to explain it.

Fast-forward a few years. I graduated, got married, and had three beautiful children. Once they went to school full time, I felt the pull back to fashion. I took styling courses in Los Angeles and

New York City, and from there worked under some amazing fashion stylists. I was blessed to make some connections . . . and the doors started opening. I styled covers of magazines, editorials, and celebrity red carpets, not to mention your everyday woman next door. My heart was full of gratitude to be able to do what I loved, as well as make people feel beautiful. But there was something I always felt was missing. I had a desire to reach more people, not just the clients I interacted with one on one. To try to connect with more women, I started a blog, which turned into a YouTube channel, and from there I was asked to be a fashion expert on TV. Which brings me to where I am today. I am so thrilled to have built a community of women I get to speak to on a regular basis through my YouTube channel.

This wonderful community asked me for a book. They take notes and rewatch the YouTube videos they love, but said they would love it if all the tips and tricks could live in one place: A book that can sit on their nightstand that they can read and reread. A book that they can give to friends as a gift. A book in which it feels like I am there with you, cheering you on, pushing your wheelbarrow, and helping you with your everyday style. Throughout these pages, I'll help you clean out your closet, create a capsule wardrobe, and get dressed with confidence. Reading this book will inspire you on your journey, and we will do it together.

My heart
was full of
gratitude to be
able to do what
I loved and
make people
feel beautiful!

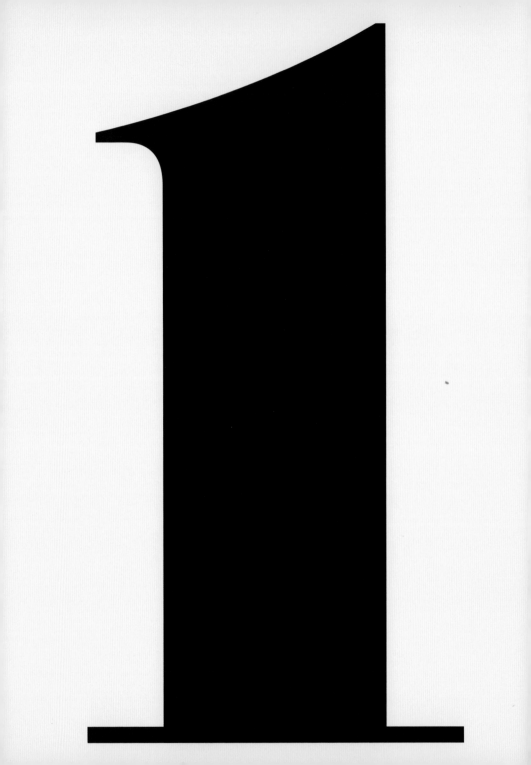

Getting Started

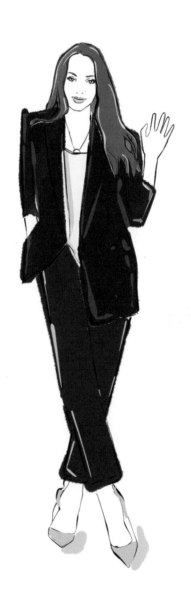

For a book that's about clothes, you might be surprised that we're going to start outside of your closet. In fact, before we even open those closet doors, we need to discover three key facts about you: your body type, your style, and your lifestyle. If you're drawn to Boho looks, your wardrobe is going to be very different from that of your preppy friend. And if your body has an apple shape, you'll look best in outfits that are different from those best suited to your pear-shaped sister. You may be drawn to leather and studs, but if you work in a corporate law office, you may have to make some compromises. When all three of these elements are considered and reflected in your wardrobe, getting dressed and feeling good will be easy. I'll guide you through this process of discovering who you are on the inside and out.

WHAT'S YOUR SHAPE?

Let me be clear: all shapes are beautiful. One body type is not better than another—they just get dressed a bit differently. Over the years, our bodies change to accommodate our lives—sometimes for beautiful reasons, sometimes for less beautiful ones. Maybe you had kids and your hips got a little wider. Or perhaps you had an illness that altered you in some way. However you've come to your current size and shape, I'd like to encourage you to love and treat yourself kindly. Yours is, after all, the only body you have, and it gets you out and about in this life.

Our eyes are drawn to balance. And that's the whole point of identifying our body type. If you're an inverted triangle—your shoulders are the widest part of you—you'll want your clothes to add volume to your lower half. Whereas a triangle (or pear) will want to add a little drama at the shoulder. If you are an hourglass, you'll want to accentuate your waist, and if you are a rectangle, you'll want to create movement, with flowing fabrics giving you some shape. My lovely circles (aka apples)—you can use asymmetrical hemlines or interesting necklines to draw the eye to whatever you feel is your best feature. To determine what your shape is, you'll need a measuring tape, a friend to help you with trickier measuring, and a full-length mirror.

I know I just said that size doesn't matter. And it's true! But we're still going to take a moment to get your current measurements, because I bet it's been a while

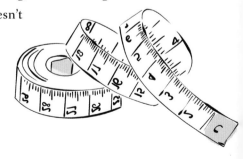

Tip: Leggings or bike shorts and a tight tank are perfect to wear for taking measurements and also for seeing your shape in the mirror.

since you've done it. Many of us have measurements in mind that are years old. Once you have your numbers, you'll be able to look at clothing sizing charts and know, with some level of accuracy, your size. Sizes can vary wildly between brands; knowing your measurements is important so you don't waste time trying to squeeze into your regular medium in a brand that makes items on the small side, meaning that you wear a large in that brand. This is particularly important when you're shopping online, where choosing the wrong size could waste your time and your money!

The Measurements You Need

→ *Height:* Stand barefoot with your back against a wall, looking straight ahead. Take this measurement from the top of your head to the floor.

→ *Shoulders:* This can be tricky, so you will need help from a friend to pull the measuring tape around you. Place the tape about 2 inches (5 cm) below your shoulder bone, stand up straight with your arms by your sides, and measure all the way around your shoulders. It's best to do this with the measuring tape right against your skin.

→ *Bust:* Put on the bra that you wear the most. Stand up and place your hands on your waist. Measure around your bust at the fullest point.

→ *Waist:* Stand up straight and place your hands on your waist. This will naturally be the narrowest part of your middle and this is where you want to measure.

→ *Hips:* Stand up straight with your hands on your waist. Measure all the way around your butt at its widest section. Here you'll definitely need assistance!

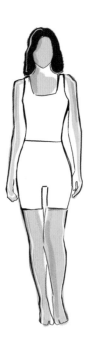

A Few Other Things to Take Note Of

→ *Neck:* Do you have a short, long, or medium neck? Standing or sitting up straight, place your hand across your neck, just under your chin. Most people will find that their four fingers cover their whole neck, from chin to clavicle. If you've got space for another finger or two (from your other hand), then you have a long neck. If you can't quite fit four fingers across your neck, you have a short neck.

→ *Shoulder slope:* Square (very straight across), standard (straight with a small slope), or sloping (smaller frame, sloping downward)?

Also, Your Proportions
+ *Balanced:* Evenly proportioned legs and torso.
+ *Short legs:* You have a long torso.
+ *Long legs:* You have a short torso.

If you need extra help, head over to my YouTube channel, where I show you how it's done. ❯ www.youtube.com/kimxo

Body Shapes

Circle: Your defining feature as an "apple" is that your tummy/ waist area has a larger circumference than your hips and shoulders. You want to draw attention away from your tummy area and to your best and most favourite assets. Pieces that work great for you have an asymmetrical hemline or deep V neckline. As well, pieces with colour blocking are fabulous for "breaking up" a tummy.

Hourglass: Your shoulders and hips are in line and your waist is smaller than both of these measurements. The best clothing for you are pieces that show off your waist. With this shape, you can really wear anything well.

Inverted Triangle: Your shoulders are wider than your hips. To create balance, you need to add weight on the bottom with full skirts or chunky boots.

Rectangle: You are long and straight, with a waist that doesn't nip in much at all. You need to add volume and create movement. Pieces with a gathered waist, a top with a scoop or V-neck, and flowing bottoms are great.

Triangle: As a "pear," you have shoulders that measure smaller than your hips. Think of balancing by adding weight, fabric, or extra detail to your shoulders. Bright tops, puffed shoulders, and ruffles are so great for you!

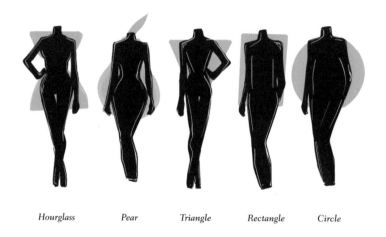

Hourglass   Pear   Triangle   Rectangle   Circle

Keep in mind that within each body type are varying sizes. There are size 0 rectangles and size 14 rectangles, for instance. You may not fit neatly into one category—you might be an hourglass with a little more curve at your hips than at your bust, say. Pick a body type you most identify with and use it as a reference moving forward.

Tip: Determining body shape is not as simple as it may sound. You are going to use the measurements you just took to get an idea of your body shape. Snap a picture of yourself in the mirror or have someone in your house snap one. Draw a straight line on the image from your shoulders to your waist to your hips and you should be able to see your shape. Is your line a curve, like the letter O? Is your line narrow at the bottom and then wider at the top like the letter V? Does your line go in and out in equal measure like the number 8? You get the picture.

WHAT'S YOUR STYLE?

When people tell me they have lost their style or can't find it, I'm reminded of the scene in *Peter Pan* where Peter thinks he's lost his shadow. He wants Wendy to help him find it and sew it back on him. Style is like Peter's shadow—you can't really lose it; your style is always with you! You may have become uninspired, but waking up the style part of yourself is easier than you might think. There are no right or wrong choices when it comes to style. It's all about finding that magic inside you, leaning into the things that make you happy.

Tip: Find your style images and save them on the platform where you spend the most time. For example, if IG is your favourite platform, every time you see a look you like, save it to a folder. Then when you go to look for inspiration, all your images are right there.

Start by paying attention to things that catch your eye. Is a flower's appealing hot pink shade something you'd love in a shirt? Do you swoon at the romanticism of Expressionist paintings? Are you drawn to anything vintage, from movies to furniture? Do clean, modern lines in architecture inspire you? These are all clues to what style choices will make you happy.

I also encourage you to look back to your childhood. Before you knew what was "cool" or trending, what did you like as a child? For me, it was wearing dresses. I thought that if my mom put me in jeans, everyone would think I was a boy. I had a pair of Buster Brown Mary Janes that I loved so much, I hated getting the bottoms dirty. To this day, I love wearing dresses, especially flowy, floral dresses.

Now let's look at some people who have their style worked out: the icons. These can be street-style stars like blogger Danielle Bernstein (who created the blog and clothing line WeWoreWhat), models like Karlie Kloss, performers like Madonna, or icons of times-gone-by like Katharine Hepburn and Brigitte Bardot. By looking at online images of stylish women and pulling together the ones you feel a style affinity for, you'll be able to narrow down your own style. Gather them up however you'd like—start a Pinterest board or Google doc, bookmark them on Instagram, or print them out and pin them to a corkboard; just put them somewhere that you can see them all at once. Give yourself time to do this, and enjoy the process. Grab a cold glass of Chardonnay, an herbal tea, coffee—whatever you fancy—then take your time and scroll away. Take a break and come back to the images later with a fresh eye.

You're looking for patterns now. What are the common threads in all the images you've chosen? Are there colours you're consistently drawn to? White collared shirts? Loafers or stilettos? Are you only choosing images of women in dresses? Or is it always denim for you? Are they sexy, tough, or sporty? Of course, lots of people are drawn to more than one style identity. You might be drawn to sexy classics, or to edgy Boho. The key is to think about what you *mostly* like. Once you have a lot of images in front of you, edit them down to the ones you really love. You may think floral dresses are kind of cute, but if they don't make you wish you were in one right now, they don't make the cut!

What you're not going to worry about right now is body type. I can hear you saying, "Well, of course Gwyneth Paltrow looks great in wide tailored pants! She's tall and thin—she can wear anything!" And you're right—she'd look great in something edgy, or Boho, but is usually dressed in classic style. We'll get to how to marry your body type with your style soon.

Style Types

Once you have your collection of images narrowed down to the ones you love most, move on to categorizing them. Of course, there are endless categories and subcategories of style, but for simplicity's sake, we're going to focus here on five style types. When you look at your favourite images, which style are they most like?

Boho

There's an earthiness to Boho style, but it's also very feminine. This style features lots of colour, flowing clothing, strappy sandals, big swinging earrings, linen shirts, and clothing made from natural materials in general. And also fabulous jewellery made with natural stones, like turquoise.

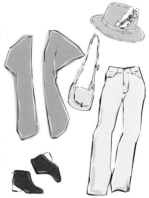

▸ *Celebrity examples:* Jane Birkin, Kate Hudson, Nicole Richie

Casual

Casual style is what we used to think of as weekend wear, but these days it can be your 24/7 look. Jeans, T-shirts, sneakers, and relaxed clothing are the backbones of casual looks.

▷ *Celebrity examples:* Jessica Alba, Jennifer Aniston, Jennifer Garner

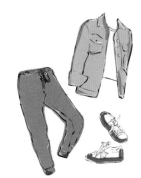

Edgy/Grunge

This category contains a variety of different looks. Grunge—with its band T-shirts, ripped jeans, and Converse sneakers—is edgy. But edgy can also be a full embrace of fashion by way of extreme proportions, bold colour, statement jewellery, and so on. In both edgy and grunge style, there's an irreverence about it that's undeniably cool.

▷ *Celebrity examples:* Miley Cyrus, Cara Delevingne, Zoë Kravitz, Rihanna, Kristen Stewart

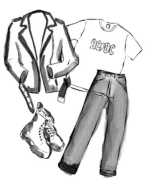

Preppy/Classic

Preppy style takes inspiration from the East Coast prep schools and sports like polo, tennis, and horseback riding. Think clean lines: white collared shirts, khaki chinos, pencil skirts, headbands, pearl or diamond earrings (though

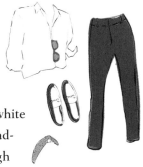
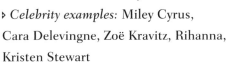

generally minimal jewellery), loafers, and fresh white sneakers.

‣ *Celebrity examples:* Carolyn Bessette-Kennedy, Gwyneth Paltrow, Kerry Washington, Reese Witherspoon, Zendaya

Sporty

Also known as athleisure, sporty style has undergone a serious upgrade over the past couple of years. No longer just meant for the gym, this style is inspired by sport but can go almost anywhere. Staples are bike shorts, big T-shirts, leggings, great sneakers, Apple watches, Swatches, and cross-body bags.

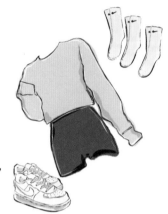

‣ *Celebrity examples:* Hailey Bieber, Bella Hadid, Kendall Jenner, Khloé Kardashian, Jennifer Lopez

YOUR LIFESTYLE

Now that you have defined your style, you have to consider taking it out into the world. Think about how you spend your time, from your work to your family time to your social life. If the Boho goddess that you have discovered in yourself has an office job, can you be yourself in your nine-to-five? The answer to this question is yes. You can add a touch of your style and personality in the office setting. For instance, you could wear a pleated midi skirt with a collared shirt, blazer, and booties (or even loafers). Even a grunge style can be made work-worthy. Imagine an oversized white blazer with the sleeves pushed up, a pair of black fitted pants, black ankle boots, and a nice fresh T-shirt underneath. An office-appropriate outfit but with a bit of a twist.

Clothes do need to be practical on some level. If you basically lived in heels until you had kids, it may be a nice to get to know the wonderful world of flats. Wearing stilettos while running after a toddler at the park may be true to your inner classic-style identity, but it may prove challenging. However, if you don't feel like giving up your heels, perhaps just pick and choose when they'll work for you. Alternatively, you can channel that vibe through jewellery or accessories.

THREE IS A MAGIC NUMBER

If you've followed me through these steps, you now have a pretty clear picture of your body type, style type, and lifestyle. The next steps are finding a way to make these three elements work together in a way that adds up to you feeling stylish and like yourself.

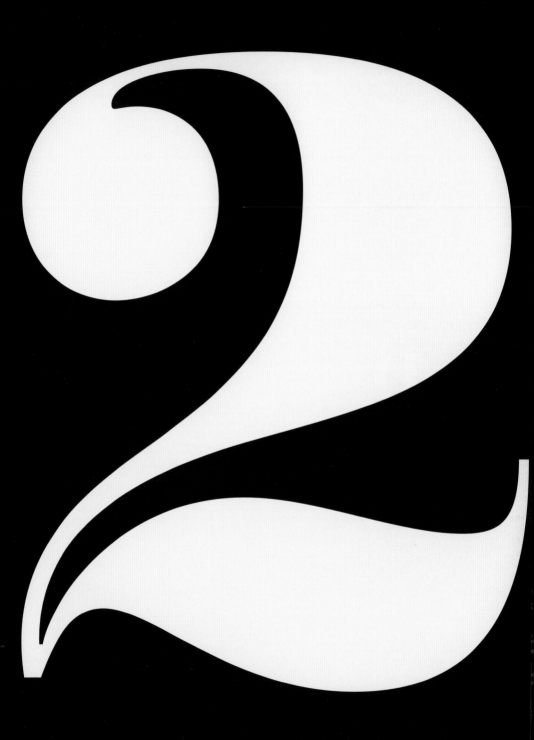

The Dragon's Lair

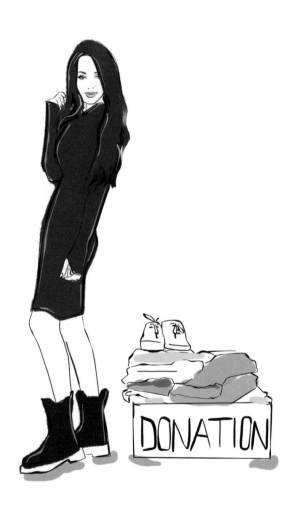

The dragon's lair, otherwise known as the clothes closet, is perhaps one of the most dreaded spots in the house. It can be a place of great pleasure when organized and filled with wonderful and well-fitting garments, and a place of great distress when it's a mess of some-fit, some-don't-fit clothes that you hide behind closed doors. How to clean it up? This chapter offers a step-by-step guide on how to get started, and tips and tricks to evaluate what should stay and what should go.

We use our clothes closet every day, yet we tend to put minimal effort into making it work for us. Anytime we need to quickly clean up our room, where does everything go? Into the closet, of course! We close those doors with a "nothing to see here" attitude and walk away, pretending there isn't an entire separate universe of energy and clothing living in there.

The closet can also be a place of avoidance. It contains old pieces of clothing that have journeyed with us through various phases of our lives, and that carries a significant amount of emotional energy. After all, there may be years' and years' worth of memories attached to those garments. But if you're not wearing them anymore and instead allowing them to take up space in your closet, they're just clutter. The hoodie you wore at the last backyard bonfire you ever had with your ex-boyfriend holds not only physical space (space you could actually use to store a beautiful new sweater) but mental and emotional space, too. Of course, many of us store clothes in other places, too, such as dresser drawers, and under-bed storage. When I talk about your "closet," I'm talking about all of it!

Dressing your beautiful body and finding your style also has lots to do with releasing what you are holding onto. You can't move forward on your style journey before cutting energetic ties to old clothing, saying a soft goodbye. You can thank the items for their time and gift them to the bonfire you make that night (good riddance to that dusty jerk), or put them into a clear garbage bag or box destined for a thrift store.

So, let's get started! Depending on how large your wardrobe is, this process could take from one hour to most of a day. Try to block off enough time to get through it in one pass. If you only get through one-quarter of your things and end up having to shove the rest back into your closet to deal with later, you may not go back to it. If organizing your closet in one pass is not possible, deal with one element at a time. For instance, go through your dresser only. Or go through everything on hangers. The main thing is to not move on to the next stage of the organizing process until you've gone through every item of clothing.

Step 1. Gather Your Materials

Things you will need:

→ Empty boxes or clear garbage bags for different
categories: keep, donate, and toss

→ Masking tape and marker for labelling

→ Notebook and pen

→ Sticky notes or stickers

→ Hangers (I prefer velvet) (See sidebar in chapter 3, page 44)

→ A friend, if you need company and a second opinion. (Just be
sure it's someone whose taste and judgment you trust.)

→ Music that puts you in a great mood

→ Full-length mirror

→ Undies, tights, or bike shorts and a tank—something you can
easily try on clothing over top of

→ Wine, coffee, tea, or water

→ Me! Pull up one of my YouTube videos of me cleaning out a
closet. I've had people who do this when they're clearing out
their closets later tell me that my videos made them feel like
I was right there with them, cheering them on.

Step 2. Step Right Up

Here's the key: just walk fearlessly toward your closet, swing
open the door, and declare yourself triumphant! Consider your
even getting to this point a full win.

Step 3. Pull It All Out

In order to organize your closet properly, it needs to be cleaned out completely. So you are going to take everything out, starting with the hanging pieces. Take everything off the rail and lay it on your bed. Now empty the shelves and drawers. For some of you, this is going to result in a huge pile of clothes. Maybe they won't even all fit on your bed and you'll have to use the floor, too. This is the moment when many people feel overwhelmed or even panicked. I've seen it a million times. Take a deep breath—this is a necessary step, and it's only going to get better from here!

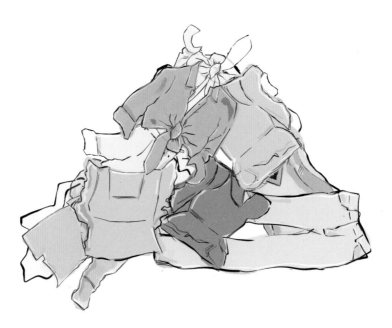

Step 4. Make Four Piles

So now you have a massive mound of clothing on your bed. First, congratulate yourself for the awesome start you've made.

Next, you're going to sort through the items, organizing them all into four piles:

1. Clothing you want to keep and is ready to go back into the closet.
2. Clothing you love and want to keep but that needs to be cleaned, mended, or tailored.
3. Clothing that is in good enough shape to donate—either to a charity or to a friend.
4. Clothing to be discarded.

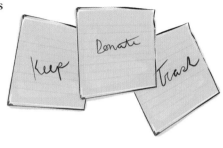

I'll share a list of places you can donate used clothing to on page 36.

How to Decide: The Rules

You're going to pick up each item of clothing and check it against the following set of rules to decide whether it stays or goes:

1. If you love it, it fits, you feel good in it, and it supports the style you're aligned with—you've got yourself a keeper!
2. If it is badly pilled, stained, or ripped, it goes. And don't take it to a thrift store! Some places—including H&M and American Eagle Outfitters—will accept damaged clothes for use in

recycled fabric. Google "recycled fabric [insert city]" to find other organizations in your area that will take unwearable clothing. Barring that, into the garbage it goes.

3. If you love it, but it's a bit stained or damaged, put it in the tailoring/cleaning pile. This also goes for items whose fit isn't quite right. Whether it's a too-long skirt or a jacket with baggy sleeves, it's always worth asking a tailor if it can be altered.

4. If you're unsure about an item, try it on. If it doesn't suit your body type (see chapter 1, page 12), it goes. You can either donate it or give it to a friend who would look fabulous in it.

5. If it's a colour you never wear but think it might be great for your next vacation, it goes.

6. If you haven't worn it for a year, try it on to remind yourself why you haven't. If it's because you don't feel good in it—it goes. If it's a piece you love and wear only for certain events, such as weddings or bar mitzvahs, it can stay. Oftentimes, our hanging on to items is grounded in fear—fear that you won't find more precious items or fear that you will lose whatever joy that item brought to you. The truth is that you are much better to release old pieces if you are not using them, and welcome new ones. Give the joy to someone else and welcome new energy! I'm not saying you can't have any sentimental items. But if even a small fraction of your wardrobe is made up of nostalgic items that don't get worn, it's time to take a deep breath and let some of them go.

7. If it holds painful memories, it goes.

Keep doing this until you have gone through everything in your wardrobe.

CLOSET STORIES

Years ago, I worked with a client who had a number of homes, and at each home there was a closet packed full of clothing from days gone by, some pieces dating back to before she was married with kids! In each of these closets were old clothes she didn't wear, and for each of those pieces there was a story about how she *may* need it and why she should keep it. These closets and old clothing weighed on her energetically—she often felt that her life was stagnant. Over the years of working together, I convinced her to donate most of these pieces. A few months after we sent off the last of the items, she called to tell me she had picked up her old love, dance, again and that her life was growing exponentially in every area. An unexplainable release! She had moved out all of the old energy, allowing for fresh space in which to grow.

Step 5. Put the Keepers Back

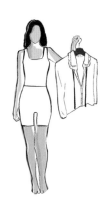

Your pile of keepers now needs to make its way back into the closet. Hang these pieces on lovely velvet hangers, or fold them up and tuck them into your dresser drawers. You'll be so glad when you're done and everything is in its rightful place!

Step 6. One Last Thing to Remember

People often keep lots of pieces on the first go-through. And don't worry—that's fine. Once you've sorted through your entire closet and put back the pieces you've decided to hold on to, you can leave it at that for a bit. After you've shopped for the new pieces you need in order to balance your wardrobe, you will likely see which of the other pieces don't belong in your closet anymore. You can then do an easier, quicker second round of purging armed with this new knowledge.

SAYING GOODBYE

Once you've accomplished the closet cleanout, you'll have a big pile of clothes you're breaking up with. Some are worn out, some just aren't right for you. But that doesn't mean they all need to end up in a landfill. One person's ill-fitting shift dress is another person's perfect LBD. I'll share ways that you can pass along clothing rather than just tossing them in the trash. But before you start physically moving pieces out of your space, take a moment to give thanks to them. Many served you well (hello, new boyfriend; hello, raise at work), and simply having the choice and ability to purchase them was a gift in itself. So many people in the world don't have the same luxury. So acknowledge your gratitude—and then get moving! Place everything into bags or boxes and label them according to where they're headed.

A WORD ON SUSTAINABILITY

The fashion industry has a disastrous impact on the environment. As fashion becomes more disposable, the situation only gets worse. I'm a fashion stylist, and I encourage women to buy new clothing where and when they need it, but I also believe in taking a thoughtful approach. Choose fewer pieces of better quality, and focus on the items you'll wear the most. And when you clear things out of your closet, sell or donate garments rather than throwing them in the garbage. Did you know that the average family in North America tosses away about 65 pounds (30 kg) of clothing each year? And only 15 percent of that gets recycled or donated—the rest ends up in landfills. Many fabrics take up to two hundred years to decompose. Thankfully, there are ways for us to do better.

The Giveaway Pile

Have another quick spin through the garments in your giveaway pile. Make a list in your notebook of the items that could or should go to specific family members or friends. Use sticky notes or stickers to label each garment with the name of the person you'll offer it to. For the rest of the items that no longer serve you, consider the many options for where to give them away. Most cit-

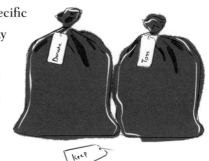

ies and towns have charity shops and organizations that help the homeless and low-income families that will gladly take your things. Some even have large bins placed around town so that you can conveniently drop off bags of clothes. Someone gets a previously owned garment, and the charity makes some money from selling it. Everybody wins! A quick online search will get you started. Search terms like "donate children's clothing [insert city]" or "donate shoes [insert city]." There are some national organizations also. Here are a few I like:

→ **American and Canadian Red Cross:** Both of these are two of the most well-respected charity organizations in North America.

→ **Dress for Success:** I personally love this one. It helps women achieve economic independence through, among other things, professional attire.

→ **Room to Grow:** This group helps parents in need of baby clothes.

- → **Value Village:** A nice option for not only clothing but other household items.
- → **Project G.L.A.M.:** A place to send fancy dresses. This group provides prom dresses to economically underprivileged teens.
- → **One Warm Coat:** An amazing organization that focuses on making sure the vulnerable keep warm with new and donated coats.
- → **Soles4Souls:** Keep your shoes out of the landfill by sending them to people who need them.
- → **thredUP:** An online consignment store where you can buy and sell.

The Selling Pile

If you've got the time and bandwidth, you may wish to sell your gently used clothes. Some outlets for this will involve a bit of effort on your part, such as eBay and Poshmark, but you have the opportunity to make some decent money on the sale. For instance, with these two platforms, you must take photos of your clothes, write a description, and then promote your listings, all on your own. Other online sites ask for less effort but take a bigger cut, such as The RealReal or brick-and-mortor consignment shops. You just send in your garments, and the staff decides on the price, and does a lot of marketing. Even fast fashion is getting in on the act, with brands like H&M providing a platform for buyers and sellers of used clothing, whether or not it's H&M's own labels.

Now that you have all your piles organized into bags or boxes, labelled, and ready to go, it's important to maintain momentum.

Remember high-school physics? An object in motion stays in motion unless acted upon by an outside force. Your clothing are the objects in motion and your procrastination the outside force. I've seen people let those bags and boxes sit in their homes for weeks! If you have a car, put them into the trunk right away. If you don't have a car, choose a spot near the front door. You want to make it uncomfortable or inconvenient to not take the next step. You won't be able to load up your car with groceries until you drop off those bags. Or you'll be tripping over the boxes at your front door until you get them out of the house.

And if you did make the switch to velvet hangers and have a pile of wire hangers, you can take them to your local dry cleaner, where they will happily take them off your hands!

Once these items are gone, take a moment to feel the lightness that comes from saying goodbye to things you don't need anymore. Good work!

CLOTHING DROP-OFF

I once had a client who drove around with bags of clothing in her car trunk for four months. They then made
their way into the back seat because she needed the
trunk space. Her car became so chaotic that she herself
felt frazzled, and that energy spread to all parts of her life!
Trust me, even if it takes all your effort and you have
other things you would rather do, take the time to drop
off the clothing at its new home. It will be worth it!

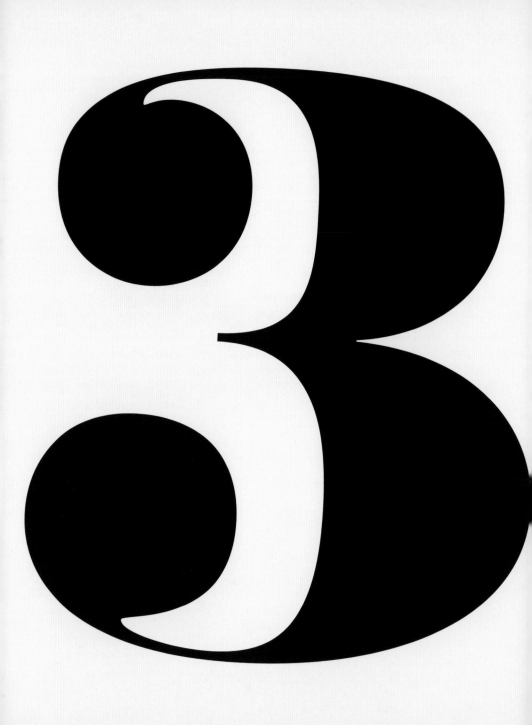

Putting It All Together

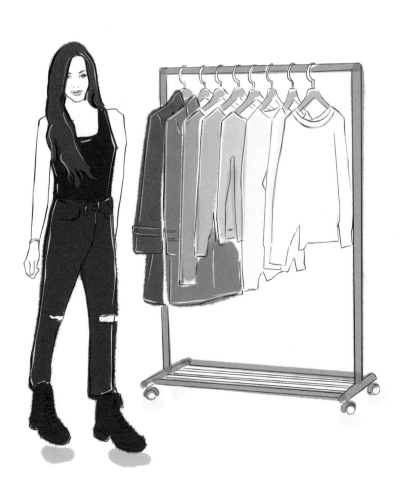

Now that you have got rid of your prom purse from 1994 and the sweater you were keeping in case you needed it for painting (real client examples), you are ready to organize your wardrobe. All your keepers are now ready to be put into drawers or onto your closet rail. My method creates a system that is pleasing to the eye and allows you to find what you're looking for with ease.

CLOSET ORGANIZATION

Most people are visually oriented, and I know from experience that people just feel better when their things are well organized. If your closet is put together in a logical way, you're going to enjoy it so much more!

A NOTE ABOUT HANGERS

I always buy velvet ones for my clients because they're gentle on clothes, and clothes stay put on them. Nothing feels more disorganized to me than a closet with wood, plastic, and bent metal hangers all smashed together. It's chaotic! I love that velvet hangers come in lots of colours, too—they add a little personality to your closet. I had hot pink ones for a while and Tiffany blue for my styling rack in my studio, and these days I have black. Part of the key to your closet feeling like a space you love is making it look as good as possible. A single colour for all of your hangers provides visual continuity and is pleasing to the eye.

First, Group by Tops and Bottoms

What I think works best for most people is to keep everything you wear on the top half of your body together on the left, and what you wear on the bottom half together on the right. If you have a two stacked bars, then shirts, blouses, and jackets go on top, and pants and skirts go on the bottom. Depending on their length, dresses and jumpsuits would hang from the higher bar.

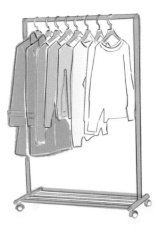

Then, Group by Colour

Keep colours together—this makes it easier to flip through quickly and scan for the right piece of clothing. Personally, I like to go light to dark, but do what works with your wardrobe.

Lastly, Group by Style or Cut

Within each colour, put similarly cut pieces together. Put all the same-coloured tanks together, T-shirts together, long sleeves together, and so on. So now when you want a white long-sleeve top, you can skip past the T-shirts and tanks and quickly find what you're looking for.

FOLDED OR HUNG?

Folded: heavy knits (hangers can really pull these out of shape), jeans, gym clothes, and casual T-shirts.

Hung: dresses, shirts, blouses, T-shirts and tanks made of more refined or delicate fabrics, jackets, and coats. If it's helpful I will actually use the hanger straps to protect the garment from stretching or to keep it on the hanger.

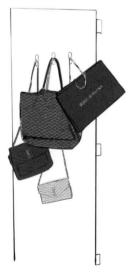

More Tips for Organizing Your Closet

➤ *Hooks:* If space permits, consider putting hooks on the back of the closet door, if that's an option. This is the spot where I hang my purses—I can see them at a glance, and I can quickly switch purses depending on what I'm wearing. You could also use this as a spot to hang a robe or long necklaces. Hooks you can screw into your closet doors are going to be the strongest, but for light items like jewellery you could use suction-cup hooks.

➤ *Jewellery drawer:* A shallow, velvet-lined jewellery

drawer is always nice to have. If your closet system or dresser doesn't have one, you can buy an insert and place it in a regular drawer. These drawers, with their various compartments, make your jewellery visible and tangle-free.

→ *Drawer dividers and bins:* These are a big deal! I use them in all my drawers. These come in various materials, from clear plastic to stiff canvas—and can be purchased at Ikea, Amazon, and lots of other organization retailers. Available in many shapes and sizes, they help keep things visible and organized. For instance, I like to separate my sport socks from all the standard black and random grey ones I have. I also separate my bras from my underwear. Long gone are the days of digging deep into the drawer abyss to find the underwear I want for the day.

Now that you are organized, it's time for something really fun . . . time to go shopping!

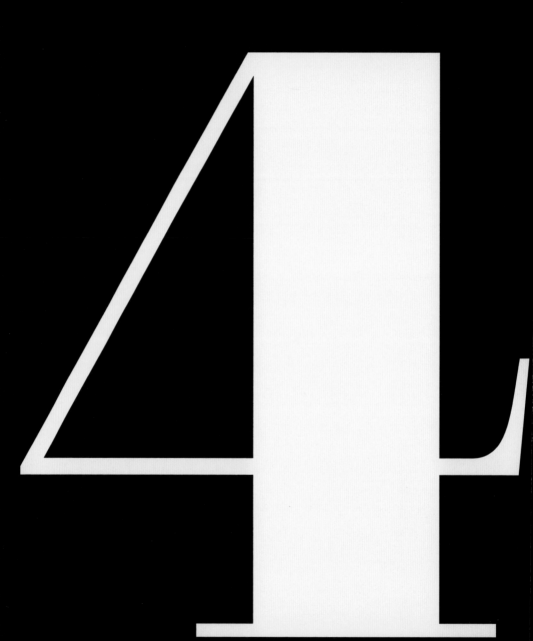

The It List

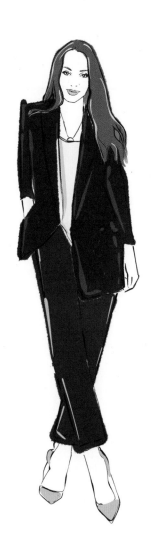

Have you ever wondered how a celebrity ends up on the it list? Or even how that one friend of yours always looks so put together regardless of the occasion? I can tell you from experience that it's because they have their style essentials nailed down. Each of those style stars—both famous and not-so-famous—have a wardrobe that works for their body, their style, and their lifestyle. And these wardrobes are made up of essentials. Maybe that sounds a little dull—but believe me, it's anything but. Your essentials—and by that I mean the ones that are right for you—are going to be the backbone of your wardrobe. They are going to show up for you time and time again and help you shine. When they've been chosen carefully, you can trust that they suit your style and your body and make getting dressed easy and fun. Knowing that the bulk of your closet is made up of great essentials allows you to play with trendier items and not feel like a fashion victim. You'll still feel like yourself in that on-trend top because you can pair it with your essential trousers and flats.

Before you get stressed out about how you don't have these items, I want to let you know it's very common not to. A few years ago, I was in New York and in the closet of a Victoria's Secret model. (Let's call her Victoria!) I arrived at her house to find the most amazing two-floor closet filled with some of the most beautiful couture pieces—and shelves and shelves of shoes. However, Victoria's biggest complaint was that she had nothing to wear. So, I started with, "Okay, let's say we are going to grab dinner after we dig into this closet—what do you have that's simple? How about a pair of dark denim jeans?" Victoria looked at me blankly and shook her head. Alright. "What about a plain black pair of booties, loafers, or white sneakers?" Again, same blank look as she shook her head no. I tried again, looking for one basic essential to build a look with. "How about a blazer?" I asked. At that point, she simply sat down on the floor and looked up at me and her beautiful closet and sighed. "Nothing. I have nothing," she said. She was right, or at least partially right: while she had a closet filled with incredible designer pieces, she needed basics to help them shine. The moral of the story is this: Don't feel bad that you don't have some of the basics. Even people who are in the fashion industry are often missing pieces of clothing that make dressing effortless.

I'm going to start by walking you through the it-list essentials (essential footwear and purses get their own chapters, chapters 5 and 6), and then we'll break it down according to body type and style.

THE EVERYDAY ESSENTIALS

Although I list several black items below, I realize that some people don't wear black. If you are very fair skinned or just don't like black, navy is a great option for you.

Tops

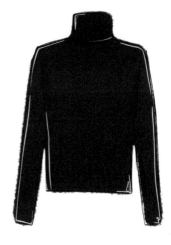

> → White T-shirts (If I find a favourite,
>   I like to have at least two or three on hand.)
> → White tanks (silk and cotton)
> → White collared dress shirt
> → Black T-shirts
> → Black tank
> → Black turtleneck
> → Black blazer (fitted and oversized)
> → Neutral cardigan (grey, navy, taupe)
> → Trench coat
> → Moto jacket
> → Wool coat
> → Puffer coat or raincoat (depending
>   on where you live)

Bottoms

+ Black dress pants: I like lightweight tapered ankle pants
+ Wool or textured pants in a more substantial fabric
+ Leather or vegan leather pants
+ Black denim
+ Navy denim
+ White denim
+ Black leggings
+ Black dressy joggers
+ Skirts (midi, pencil, mini—depending on your body type)

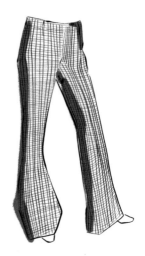

All Over

+ Day dresses: Dark knee-length dress that can take you from a meeting to dinner.
+ Cocktail dresses: Knee-length or a bit longer in either a light, soft fabric or a fabric with body and shine. You should have one black and then if you add more you can consider colours or patterns.
+ Jumpsuits: For those who don't love wearing dresses, jumpsuits can be a good alternative. You get that one-and-done-feeling with a lot of comfort.

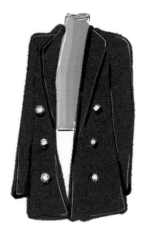

If you had only the items listed, you could put together a lot of killer outfits. For instance, the black turtleneck, leather pants, and oversized blazer looks super on a date, the same black turtleneck with black dress pants is perfect for the office, and that black turtleneck paired with white denim looks sharp for brunch with friends. Of course, these are likely not all the items you have in your wardrobe. These essentials will pair with any non-essential items you have— and honestly, they will probably make them look even better. Do you have a colourfully printed blouse that always feels like it's a bit much? Pair it with dark denim to tone it down. Or maybe you have a cute novelty T-shirt that you've never figured out how to wear. Pull your black blazer over it and it will feel fresh (not silly).

ESSENTIALS BY BODY TYPE

Not every person will have the same "essentials." The key to feeling great every day is having the essentials that are right for *you*. Below, I suggest the basics for the various body types. Check out the charts I've created for a quick reference on page 129.

Circle

You want clothes that skim the body. Whether you're wearing a flowy jersey fabric or a crisp cotton, you want pieces that are not tight, not loose, not because you've got anything to hide, but because it will give you the longest silhouette. Longer tops and jackets work well, rather than ones that stop at the waist. Deep V-necklines and short or pushed-up sleeves are great ways to show off some skin. Swingy tunics with angled hemlines—either shorter in the front and longer in the back or asymmetric with one side longer than the other—are flattering because they keep your torso from looking boxy. Look for jeans and trousers with a boot cut or flare.

Hourglass

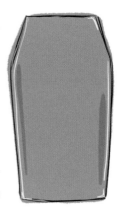

You can wear most things, but put the focus on your waist. Choose tops that are fitted and structured, like wrap or belted tops. A classic moto jacket is a fabulous piece, as it is often cut right to the waist. Cropped blazers that land above your hips are perfect, too. High-waisted trousers and jeans, and slim pencil skirts, suit an hourglass figure. Loose, flowy blouses or skirts can look a little sloppy on this body type.

Inverted Triangle

When your shoulders are broad, you want to keep your tops simple. So, no big shoulder pads, no puffed shoulders or sleeves, and generally not a lot of frou-frou above your waist. A tee with a deep V-neckline will draw the eye downward. Choose pants and skirts with movement and flow. You want to add volume at the bottom with A-line skirts, ruffles, or peplums, and wide-leg trousers.

Rectangle

Look for pieces that flow and create curves where you may not have a lot. For on top, invest in wrap blazers and silk blouses that hang softly. Deep V- or sweetheart necklines are ideal for highlighting your neck and collarbone. Dresses and tops with a peplum will add curve to your silhouette. You'll look great in bottoms and skirts with volume, such as pleated skirts and printed or textured pants. Fit and flare dresses will define your waist and add a little flounce.

Triangle

You want to emphasize your beautiful shoulders with detailed, ruffle, or puff sleeves. Blazers with definition—either by way of shoulder pads or just a seam that sits exactly at the shoulder, rather than a drop shoulder—will add volume and balance out your hips. You can even find T-shirts these days that have shoulder pads or are cut to exaggerate your shoulder line. You can layer a shoulder-padded T-shirt under a sweater to get a soft but defined silhouette. Jackets that hit at your waist will highlight your upper body. For the bottom, choose simple and slim skirts and pants, rather than anything with a lot of volume or flourish at the hem.

ESSENTIALS BY STYLE TYPE

I believe that everyone needs wardrobe essentials regardless of their personal style. To make those essentials work, you need to find the right ones for you. As Audrey Hepburn said, "There is a shade of red lipstick for every woman." This holds for essentials and personal style, too: there is a blazer or jean cut that's just right for you and that will fit your personal style (which you learned about in chapter 1).

Boho

Boho women are modern hippies—they love flowy dresses and big, soft hats, and they would live in sandals year round if that were practical. Fabric is key to this style, and if you love this vibe, you'll be drawn to natural fibres like cotton, linen, leather, suede, silk, velvet, and cork. The variety of textures that come

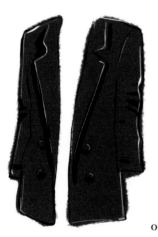

from these textiles is what you love. And while you're not afraid of colour or pattern, you may tend toward slightly muted hues. Yes, you still need a blazer, but yours will be very different from your preppy friend's version. Yours will be less structured and might have a shawl collar. You like short and long skirts and dresses, but they always flow, never squeeze. Your white shirt will have some texture to it. Your denim is soft, not stiff, whether it's a skinny cut or full-on flares. You get glam from beading, tassels, hats, embroidery, and rustic jewellery. One of your outerwear pieces of choice in the spring and fall is a loose, kimono-like coat.

Casual

You like to keep it real in life. You want to be comfortable and still look great. There are essentials out there for you, too. Your blazers might be made of terry cloth. Or you opt for a belted cardigan over a relaxed jersey white collared shirt. Your bottom might be a long grey sweater skirt or a relaxed pair of jeans. You love flat boots, loafers, and sneakers. To keep things from getting too basic, add jewellery, like a chain-link necklace, a chunky belt, or a hair accessory such as a scrunchie or a headband. I recommend paying extra attention to quality and the condition of your casual favourites to avoid looking schlumpy. There's a world of difference between a fresh white T-shirt in a good-quality cotton and the fun-run T-shirt that's been kicking around your closet for 10 years! Casual outerwear for you includes a denim jacket for spring and summer and a cozy wrap wool coat or fluffy teddy coat in a neutral colour for the winter.

Edgy/Grunge

If your style is edgy, your essentials will be pushed in some way. You need essentials as much as any other style type, but they're never basic. Maybe it's the silhouette—your blazer is oversized or very nipped in at the waist, and your trousers might be cropped or sculpted. The knitwear you're drawn to has interesting details, like a cocoon silhouette or slits at the elbow. If you're on the grungy end of the spectrum, you'll gravitate toward mostly black and white, while those on the edgy end might be drawn to hits of super-saturated colours. You're also drawn to contrasts when it comes to texture— you love to pair a tweedy coat with studded boots. The outerwear of choice is your leather moto jacket and a cool, oversized wool coat.

Preppy/Classic

If you are a fan of Carolyn Bessette-Kennedy or Jackie O, you love the essentials in their most pure and classic form. You feel great in a crisp white collared shirt, paired with a single-breasted fitted blazer that hits at the waist, dark-navy skinny jeans, a pair of black pumps, and a structured tote. Pencil skirts or simple shift dresses are better for you than anything too frilly. Your outerwear is a classic trench in the spring and a camel-coloured alpaca coat in the winter. You love colour mixed in with your black and whites and add it to your wardrobe via sweaters, T-shirts, baseball caps, belts, and footwear. You're not one for a lot of texture in fabrics and prefer smooth cotton poplin, tropical wools, and fine-knit cashmere.

Sporty

If you are the sporty type, the explosion of athleisure on the market is the best thing that ever happened to you. You love the comfort of pieces like hoodies and joggers, but they also have a practicality that speaks to your lifestyle. It's important to keep things clean and elevated or this look can get sloppy in a hurry (sporty doesn't mean a worn-out T-shirt and sweats). A double-breasted oversized blazer over a hoodie, paired with vegan leggings and dressed-up sneakers, is your take on an essential outfit. Finish with a cross-body bag in black, perhaps with a designer baseball cap, and you're both stylish and practical. Your outerwear of choice could be a mid-weight, quilted, long bomber or a long sleeveless puffer vest that you can wear over your hoodie or long-sleeve shirt.

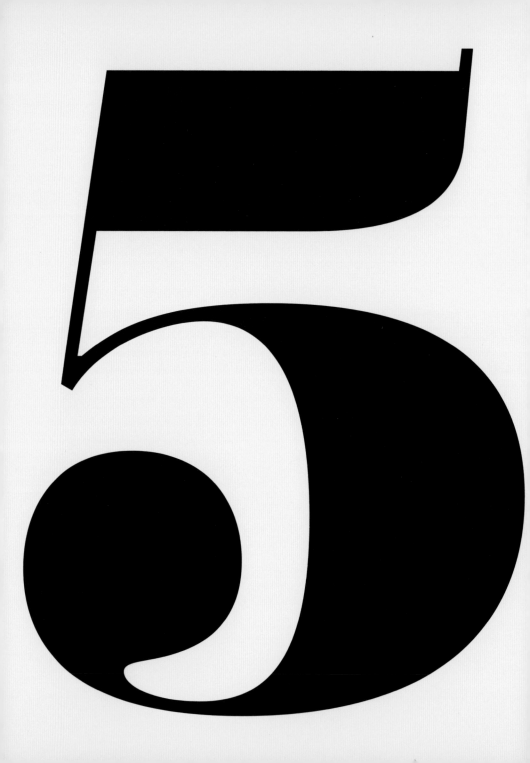

Essential
Footwear

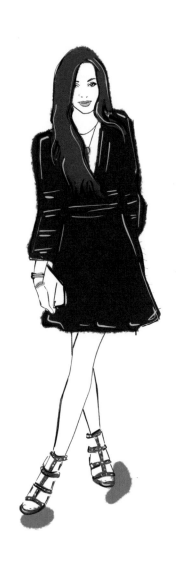

Footwear can make or break an outfit. In fact, if an outfit is feeling a bit off, always start by switching out your shoes. The key is to have shoes that suit your style and balance your body type. So, although there is a basic list of essential shoes, every body and style type will have their own list (see my style charts on page 129). As well as exploring essential footwear for every body and style, we'll look at where to spend and save, and how to look after your shoes so that they last.

Basic Shoe Wardrobe

- ✦ Neutral (black or tan) booties
- ✦ Combat/flat boots
- ✦ Tall boots

+ White sneakers
+ Black pumps
+ Neutral-coloured pumps
+ Flats (like ballet slippers or loafers)
+ Flat leather sandals
+ Open-toe strappy sandals (heeled and flat)
+ Rubber flip-flops (for pool or beach)
+ Workout sneakers

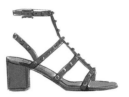

FOOTWEAR BY BODY TYPE

Circle

You beautiful "apples" are widest in your middle, and usually your best feature are your legs. The best thing you can do is draw attention to your legs—fun, exciting, and dramatic shoes are right up your alley! With that, stilettos will be your best friend, as well as shoes with interesting colours and eye-catching details.

Hourglass

You have a beautiful shape, generous bosom, derriere, and an accentuated waistline. Avoid anything overly clunky or delicately dainty that will take away from your balanced frame. You look fabulous in any sky-high heel—but I love the peep toe for you. Wedge boots and sandals look super on you as well. Avoid anything clunky that takes attention away from your balanced fame.

Inverted Triangle

Those with an inverted triangle body type (wider on the top than the bottom) look good with a heavier shoe or boot, something that balances out their top half. Chunky loafers, sneakers with a bigger sole, combat boots, and heels with some weight or embellishment are perfect for you. Stay away from really dainty versions of these basics or you will feel very top-heavy.

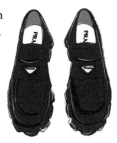

Rectangle

The body silhouette with the least curves can be balanced and feel smoother with simple feminine versions of the classic shoes. Pumps, loafers, and sneakers with an almond or round toe will help you appear softer and more curvy. You want to avoid an ultra pointy shoe, as it will elongate your frame and emphasize the linear lines.

Triangle

Your hips are your widest point, and you may also have heavier ankles and fuller legs, so you want to draw attention upward. Stick to neutral-coloured shoes, open-toe wedges, and heeled sneakers (their volume is vertical, not horizontal). Avoid anything too chunky (like a heavy platform), tall boots that are too tight around the calf, or gladiator sandals that will draw attention to your bottom half.

FOOTWEAR BY STYLE

Because shoes add so much to a look, your essential footwear will be guided by your style. Pointy-toed stilettos may look good on your body type, but if your style is sporty, they're not going to feel right for you.

Boho

Just as with your clothing, Boho dressers will be drawn to texture in their footwear—suede, velvet, fringe, and tassels. In the cooler months, you like cowboy boots or riding boots; in warmer months, you like not-too refined sandals—like gladiators or fishermen style, or fabric espadrilles. You gravitate toward neutral colours, but some hits of colour and metallic totally suit your vibe.

Casual

To go with your casual wardrobe, you go for sneakers, slip-on flats, and pull-on ankle boots. Sneakers with dresses and skirts are a perfect combination for you. When getting dressed up, you're more comfortable in a low or kitten heel.

Edgy/Grunge

Women on the grunge end of the spectrum will live in black shoes and boots, preferably with buckles and studs and a chunky tread. On the edgy end of things, you like exaggerated shapes like pointy or squared-off toes, colourful leather or suede, and details like fringe or mesh.

Preppy/Classic

Classics—from ballet flats to simple pumps to lace-up Oxfords or loafers—are in your wheelhouse. Your boots are classic English riding style or clean ankle booties. You tend to like shoes and boots in smooth leather or suede rather than in materials with a lot of texture or decorative details. Your casual shoes are white canvas sneakers or simple sandals.

Sporty

Sneakers are an obvious go-to for you. In fact, you probably have a collection of them—some for working out, some for casual wear, and even some heeled ones for going out. For winter, you prefer a slightly chunky ankle boot, and in the warmer months, you like an athletic slide. Try adding heels to your more refined joggers for an evening look.

TO MATCH OR NOT TO MATCH?

I get asked this question often, and my answer is always the same: I love matching purses and shoes. Matching comes in and goes out of trend; however, I think it can pull a look together. If your look isn't exactly as finessed as you'd like it to be, some repetition will make it feel balanced.

SHOPPING FOR SHOES

Over the years, I've amassed useful tips for shoe shopping. Here are a few things you'll want to keep in mind before you hit the stores:

→ *Choose your timing.* Always go shoe shopping in the afternoon, as your feet will have expanded from your morning's activities. You'll be glad for that extra comfort and space in the shoe you end up purchasing.

→ *Prioritize comfort.* If you have wide feet, don't try squeezing them into narrow pumps; if you have flat feet, avoid shoes with a built-in arch that are going to create a dull ache as you walk. If you're not comfortable, it's going to show up in your body language, and even the best outfit will look off. Or you'll just never wear them (and you will have wasted your money).

→ *Dress right.* Wear the kind of socks or tights you'll wear with your shoes. Don't wear sweat socks when you're looking for sexy stilettos!

→ *Get up.* Make sure you try on both shoes in a pair and stand up and walk. Your feet expand when you stand, and you need the full experience of the shoes.

→ *Get thrifty.* Don't be afraid to shop at high-end consignment stores. There are often gems in there that have never been worn.

→ *Buy the dupe.* Save on trendy shoes that you won't spend that much time in, like a hot-pink pump that you need for one event to match a dress or when a trend like massive chains on the shoe is in . . . buy a dupe!

→ *Consider colour.* Particularly for those of you who wear a lot of black or other neutrals, a coloured shoe is an easy way to add interest to an outfit. Same goes for metallics.

→ *Practise brand loyalty.* Shoe brands will often use the same lasts (the foot-shaped moulds that shoemakers work with) over and over again. When you find a brand with a good fit for you, stick with them!

→ *Buy what you truly love.* Take your time finding the right pair of shoes. I suggest buying the best quality that you can afford—particularly when it comes to classics, like ballet flats and pumps. Not only will they be more comfortable, but a high-quality pair of shoes can last a lifetime if they are taken care of properly. (I still have a pair of my mother's in my closet.)

CARING FOR YOUR SHOES

Over the years, I have destroyed very expensive designer shoes—sometimes because of ignorance and sometimes because of impatience. There was a time when I didn't know that I should give my leather shoes the same protective spray that I use for suede ones. And I've been so eager to wear a pair of suede heels that I didn't take the time to spray them, and they got ruined in the rain. Either way, I learned the hard way, and I know now that if you are going to invest money in shoes that you want to last for decades, you must take care of them.

↪ *Shoe repair.* Start by getting to know a cobbler in your area. This is someone who can resole your shoes, polish them, replace your lifts (those little rubber bits on the tip of the heels), and ultimately extend the life of your shoes. A really good shoe-repair person can work wonders.

↪ *Prep.* Before I wear shoes or boots out of the house, I do a little prep work. I always use a waterproof spray on suede or leather shoes. You'll want to repeat this step once or twice a year, depending on the weather where you live. Check the bottom of your shoes—oftentimes the soles of high-quality shoes are made of leather, which quickly deteriorates with wear. I take these to a shoe-repair person and ask them to add a thin rubber layer to the soles. It's inexpensive and makes a big difference!

↪ *Cleanup.* Give shoes and boots a quick wipe before you put them away at the end of the day and they'll always be ready to go when you reach for them the next time.

↪ *Shapers.* Shoe and boot inserts help your footwear—particularly those made of leather and suede—keep their shape. They come in different shapes for different kinds of shoes and are made of plastic or wood. The plastic type is less expensive, but wood absorbs moisture and odour. Pop the forms into your shoes or boots as soon as you take them off, while they're still warm. After 24 hours, you can remove the forms from your shoes (and potentially use them for other shoes), if you like, but boot forms should always be left in when you're not wearing the boots, to stop them from flopping over and creasing.

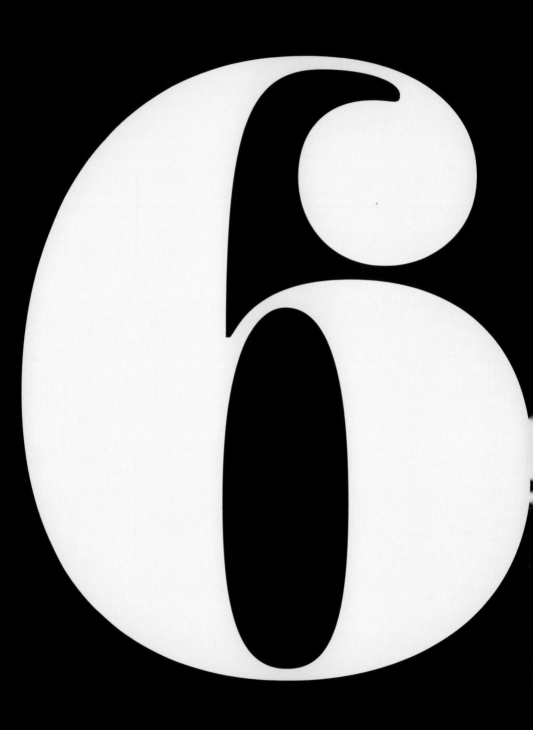

Essential
Purses

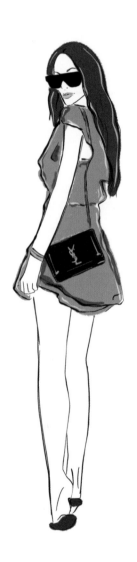

Many of us don't often spend much time thinking about our purses. We tend to carry around the same ratty tote we've used for years. And besides that functional tote, we have a bunch of random clutches and small purses sitting at the back of our closet that we bought at the 11th hour for an event to match an outfit. But there are a few essential purses that will really make your outfits and which you will be grateful you have. It's not important to have the latest trendy purse, but rather, one that suits your body type and style. In this chapter, I explain which bags look best with each, how to use your bags to complement your outfits, and how to choose colours that are right for your skin tone, as well as basic maintenance and upkeep.

In my opinion, it's important to take your time shopping for purses, and then purchasing the best-quality and most classic version you can afford. Less is more here—I'd rather you invest in fewer good-quality bags than have lots of cheap ones. And when you are spending more money, it's best to stick to neutral colours, which can easily transition and be paired with many outfits. The examples I give below are designer so that you can look them up online or in a boutique and imagine their size and shape, but there are lots of options at other price points. For instance, you'll often find good-quality, great-looking bags at vintage or consignment shops for a fraction of what they cost new.

ESSENTIAL BAGS

Tote

The tote is a key element of any wardrobe. It's practical and roomy. It's handy for carrying work papers and a computer, plus your makeup bag and kids' belongings. A tote is my favourite airplane bag. It's often stuffed full with my neck pillow, books, and smaller wallet on a chain when I am travelling. You can find totes in cotton, canvas, leather, or vegan leather. Because this is an everyday bag, look for a sturdy material that can be spot-cleaned easily. For years, I had a coated canvas tote, which saw me through three kids and hundreds of flights, and made its way to multiple sets full of styling tools. I liked that I could sit it down anywhere and never worry about staining the bottom, and I could easily wipe it down with any cloth (including the occasional wet wipe!). After about 10 years, I bought a Goyard tote in a similar size. It is still my current go-to large bag. I believe it's important to invest in the best quality you can afford. Both these totes, while on the pricier side, have lasted me a good 10 years each and they are a classy touch to any outfit.

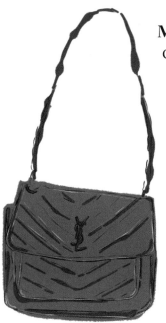

Medium Cross-Body

Cross-body bags are the perfect combination of compact and versatility. Choose this style when you're on the go and want minimal fuss. I get a lot of use from it when I am working (pulling clothing for photo shoots), on vacation, and also when my look is quite casual. I only have one; it's black and indestructible. I have had the YSL Niki bag in crinkled vintage leather. I like this bag for two reasons: first, the leather is not easily stained (I'm sure you are starting to see a theme here), and second, it has a convertible chain strap, so I can wear it cross-body when I need my hands free, or on the shoulder for another style when I want a different look. It's big enough to carry everything I need in the course of a day but not so big that I'm weighed down.

The Dressy Handbag

This is a handbag every woman should own. We all need one go-to dressy bag that goes everywhere, from dinner out to a fancy party. Whether it comes with a shoulder strap or a top handle, this bag is smaller than a tote but larger than a clutch—it only needs to hold your phone, your credit card, and a lipstick. I love my YSL Medium Kate in beige with a gold chain strap. It's structured, it's classy, and it looks intentional with everything I pair it

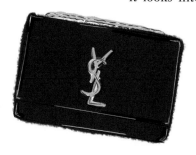

with. The dressy-handbag category has a huge amount of variety. If you're only going to have one such bag, I'd choose black, maybe with a little sparkle or decorative flourish.

The Clutch

A clutch is a small purse we carry in our hand, under the arm, or on our shoulder. It's almost always an evening bag and needs to be big enough only for your keys, your credit card, and a lipstick. Because it gets the least use (by most of us), this bag often gets forgotten. I feel like most women panic-buy clutches when they have an event or special occasion. Don't do it! Often, having one clutch is enough, but it is important to choose wisely. It's ideal if it's simple and goes with all your evening looks. If you don't love the idea of having to hold a clutch all night long, look for versions with chains—either shoulder or wrist length. I have purchased the iconic Chanel half moon wallet on a (silver) chain, and it has been in use for over 15 years! What I love about it is the textured leather (it doesn't scratch), the unique shape, and how it holds my phone and a lipstick, plus has slots for a few cards. Other classic high-quality clutches and shapes that are good to look at for reference are the YSL wallet on a chain and the Bottega Veneta pouch.

BAGS BY BODY TYPE

Have you ever been faced with that moment when, having coveted a certain bag, you trek to the store, only to realize that it just doesn't suit you? The truth of the matter is that, like many other fashionable items, bag suitability boils down to body type. If it's balance that we're always looking for, then it makes sense that bags are a part of our overall visual. Like everything else, it's all about proportions!

Circle

As an "apple," your waist is the widest part of your body; you may or may not have a big bust. To de-emphasize the midsection, choose structured or boxy bags with short straps you hold in your hand. Avoid big floppy bags and cross-body bags that sit at your waist. Also, small bags are not the best choice because they make you look larger than you are. Styles such as the Celine 16 Bag or Gucci's bowler-style Ophidia are amazing options for you!

Hourglass

The hourglass beauties are blessed because, generally, you can wear most purses. The only direction I would give you is to watch for proportion—you don't want your bag to overwhelm you. You want to draw attention to your waist.

Inverted Triangle

Because your shoulders are broader than your waist, you want to add volume and weight to your lower half. Bags for you are any with a longer strap so they sit on your hip, or belt bags that sit on your hip. You want to avoid clutches or bags with short straps.

Rectangle

Given your athletic body type, you are mostly straight up and down, so create balance by creating the illusion of curves. You want a softer bag, made of pliable leather or suede, and an unstructured clutch that tucks under your arm.

Triangle

You beautiful "pears" are curvier in the bottom half of your body, so aim for bags that emphasize the upper half of your body. Bags that are perfect for you are ones that fall between the waist and hips. Bags that go across the body work well as long as they hit higher. Something like Prada's nylon studded belt bag would be ideal if worn across the body, as it adds attention on the top half of you. Avoid slouchy and small bags, as well as those that fall on your hip.

BAGS BY STYLE

Boho

Bags with some texture—linen, suede, or pebbled leather—will appeal to a Boho gal. You're also drawn to fringe, tassels, and embroidery. You go for browns, tans, or soft colours over harsh black.

Casual

You love canvas totes for the summer, and pebbled leather or suede all year round.

Edgy/Grunge

Women with an edgy style will go for quirky shapes and textures. Grunge girls will be drawn to black leather, often with buckles or studs.

Preppy/Classic

Your day bags are either smooth leather or canvas, and for evening you like patent leather or satin. You gravitate to black, navy, or tan.

Sporty

Nylon is your fabric of choice, though you like a leather cross-body, too. A leather or nylon backpack can double as a day bag for you.

Like everything else, it's all about proportions!

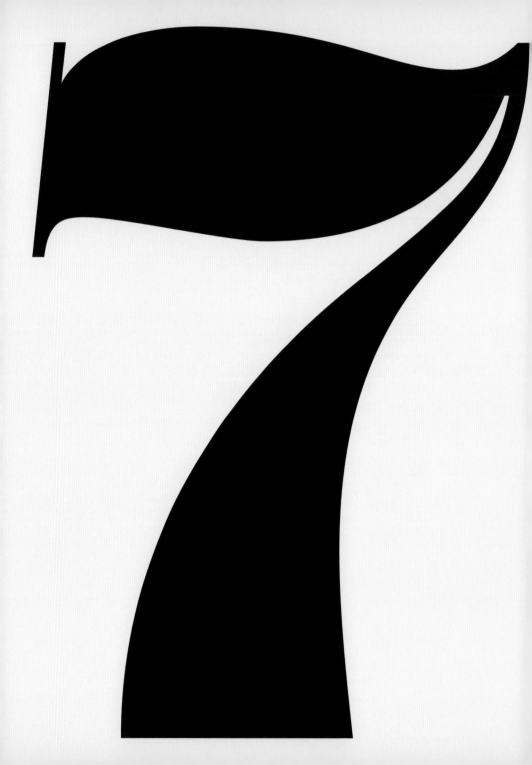

Essential
Accessories

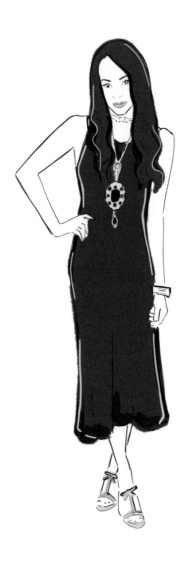

Once you have a clean and organized closet, and you have thrown on a crisp white shirt and midi skirt, along with cute sneakers and a cross-body bag, what are the finishing touches? How do those women who always look fantastic pull it off? What's their secret? Oftentimes, the key to looking fabulous and feeling good is in the finishing details. A pair of gold hoops, a few delicate gold necklaces, and a ring can go a long way. When you need to tie your hair back in the middle of the day, are you using a grungy elastic or are you pulling a brightly coloured silk scrunchie out of your bag and securing your locks with style? In this chapter, I share a list of my personal favourite outfit finishers and also list suggestions for outfit finishers according to body type and style.

Trust me, there is gorgeous jewellery out there for everyone.

ESSENTIAL JEWELLERY

A note about budgets: the price range of jewellery is vast. You can pick up pieces for a song or invest in fine jewellery at eyewatering prices. Trust me, there is gorgeous jewellery out there for everyone. If I mention diamonds, know that you can find classy-looking cubic zirconia versions for a fraction of the price. When I suggest gold, it can be gold-plated pieces rather than solid gold. When it comes to jewellery, you may want to consider looking at vintage or consignment shops to find deals. Plus, there are lots of brands on the market now making quality, stylish jewellery at reasonable prices.

Diamonds

Studs

You can't go wrong with a pair of diamond studs. They are perfect for day or night, casual or dressy looks, in summer or winter. They can be worn on their own and also with other jewellery. Before I bought my first real pair, I wore the best pair I could afford; they were crystal set in gold—they looked elegant and I felt beautiful in them. Since some semi-precious stones can lose their lustre over time, you might have to buy a second pair. If you're able to save up for a pair of real diamond studs, even if small, know that they will last a lifetime. They'll never go out of style, and putting them on will add style even to your jeans–and–T-shirt looks.

Tennis bracelet and necklace

These are simple, pliable narrow strings of symmetrical diamonds on a thin chain. The bracelet is named for American tennis star Chris Everet, who was known for wearing an inline diamond bracelet on the court. The tennis bracelet and necklace are some of my favourite pieces of fine jewellery, and I have acquired them both over time as special gifts—I wear them all the time! I tell my clients to do the same with all their special pieces: if you love it, wear it. The nice thing about a tennis necklace is that it can be worn alone as a special piece with a dress, or layered. I wear mine layered with my everyday "K" (for "Kim") necklace. You can mix metals, so whatever the setting of your tennis necklace or bracelet, feel free to mix it with other pieces. I wear my tennis necklace at the beach, by the pool on holidays, at special dinners . . . and every day!

Metals

Hoops

Hoops, in white or yellow gold, silver or sterling, are another basic that never goes out of style. The style and size of the hoops may change with trends, but hoops themselves stand the test of time and are a very easy way to add subtle glamour to your look. A discreet hoop will look timeless on those with a classic or casual style. A chunkier, textured hoop will suit an edgy style. A larger hoop dresses up athletes, and Boho girls can go to town with shoulder-grazing hoops.

Chains

Even if you are not a jewellery person, having one fine yellow or white gold or silver necklace can really help you look put together because of the way it adds a subtle extra layer to an outfit. I suggest gold or white gold because it won't tarnish, and if you don't like to fuss with jewellery, you can leave it on 24/7. I never take off my gold necklace, which makes my life easier—I even wear it in the shower and pool, and at the gym, and it adds a little sparkle. Another trick is to layer it with a second or third fine necklace. I think the reason this look is so intriguing is that *you*, not a jewellery designer, put it together. Depending on how many necklaces you have, you can change up the combinations to suit your mood and outfit. It adds a bit of interest to your look without weighing you down. It's nice to have a few at varying lengths, so that you can choose depending on the neckline of your shirt or dress. While I love the look of a simple chain, I also love the look of pendants or charms on chains for the personal touch they add to outfits.

Bracelets, bangles, and cuffs

Gold, silver, or platinum bangles, which are simple, circular brace-lets, look great alone or stacked in multiples. They can be very simple or stamped with designs. Chain-link bracelets give a similar effect to bangles but are more flexible on your wrist. Many chain bracelets allow you to add charms. A cuff is a wider, solid bracelet with an opening to slip your wrist into. These usually shape to your arm and sometimes come painted or enamelled.

CHUNKY NECKLACES

When choosing a heavier necklace, take note of your neck length. If you have a shorter neck, you'll want to choose a piece with some length to create the illusion of a longer neck. Chokers and bib necklaces may not be the best for you. Stick to necklaces that elongate.

Fine Gold

Fine gold jewellery is doubly special: it's beautiful and also tends to be associated with significant moments. Wedding bands come to mind, but it could also be in the form of a simple chain necklace that was an anniversary gift, or a bracelet you inherited from your grandmother. Because they tell a story, these sentimental pieces really add to your personal style like no other pieces can. Since gold is expensive, it's best to go with simple, classic styles rather than trendy shapes (unless price is no object, in which case, lucky you!).

Pearls

Earrings
Pearls have the distinction of being the oldest gemstone known to humans. There are so many beautiful versions of pearl earrings that you are by no means confined to classic pearl studs. You can find beautiful pearls on delicate hoops or a double drop earring, for instance. Pearls are classic and versatile, and can be mixed with other jewellery.

Necklaces
Pearl necklaces are definitely a classic—but depending on the length of the strand and the size of the pearls, they can come off differently. A strand of small pearls that sits on your collarbone lends a delicately feminine look, while a double strand of gumball-sized pearls makes a bold impression. Pearls look beautiful against jewel-tone colours and also with a white tee.

Costume Jewellery
Costume jewellery is a fun and inexpensive way to add character to your look. The trend of the chunky necklace comes and goes, but if it suits your style, it's always a good addition to your wardrobe. And

it can be any type of statement necklace, anything from a beautiful turquoise layered piece to strands of pearls to a big, heavy gold chain. Also, be on the lookout for brooches, bangles, clip-on earrings, and even decorative hair pins.

Watches

Watches are a very personal thing. With everything from our ovens and cars to our phones and computers telling us the time, watches are not really necessary anymore and are more of a style statement than anything. Watches tend to be a big thing for men because, as I often hear, it may be the only "jewellery" they wear.

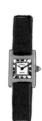

A CLASSIC WATCH

The Cartier Tank watch is one of my favourite classics, worn by many famous celebrities and artists over the years, including Princess Diana and Jackie O. Fun fact: the design on the inside of the numbers was meant to symbolize a railroad track and inspire travel.

ESSENTIAL HATS

Hats are an overlooked accessory that can add so much to a look. They have a function, obviously, but they are also just one more opportunity to show off your style. Depending on where you live, your hat requirements will vary. If you live in Palm Beach, you most likely won't have a big selection of toques, but you likely have hats that block the sun. That being said, I'll share with you a few of my favourite styles, and you can adapt for climate:

- Baseball cap
- Matador
- Panama
- Straw hat
- Toque
- Visor

HAIR ACCESSORIES

How many of you wear a black hair elastic around your wrist just in case of emergency? I am going to go out on a limb here and suggest that that elastic is, in fact, *not* an accessory. There are so many fabulous hair accessories out there, so why not shake things up a little and add one or two to your repertoire? I love fabric scrunchies, as they add softness and colour to a ponytail. Headbands are a chic way of keeping hair out of the face and can also add colour, texture, and a bit of volume to your look.

BELTS

I suggest having a few classic belts in different widths and colours in your closet. Not every pair of trousers with belt loops needs a belt each and every time—but a belt *can* add a layer to your outfit. Don't be afraid to replace the belt that comes with a dress or pants with your own leather one to change up the look. (And, if you have an hourglass shape, belts are often one of your best accessories, as they highlight your waist and emphasize one of your best features. Lucky you!)

SCARVES

Depending on where you live, you may want to have a few scarves of varying weights to add functionality and style to outfits. A large, square silk scarf can be folded or rolled into several different shapes, for different looks. Drape it under the lapel of your jacket or coat, knot one snugly under the open collar of a white button-up shirt, wear it bandana style to fill in a V-neck of a sweater, tie it to the handle of your handbag . . . the list of possibilities is virtually endless. A large, woolly scarf can be tucked inside your winter coat or draped around the shoulders of your winter coat.

ACCESSORIES BY STYLE

Boho

If you are Boho, chances are you are going to lean into a wide-brim fedora or a beautiful matador. For a festival-ready look, pair your fedora with a bright tunic layered with funky necklaces and some turquoise-encrusted cuffs and you are ready to enjoy the moment in style. Pair a floppy straw hat with a flowing dress and colourful dangling earrings and you will look like you sauntered right out of a magazine!

Casual

Casual gals like to keep things simple. You like a simple gold or silver necklace, small stud earrings and a watch without too many

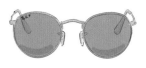

bells and whistles. You dress up your white T-shirt and jeans with a cute toque and a thin scarf wrapped around your neck.

Edgy/Grunge

There are so many vintage baseball caps that look cool—throw one of those on and let your hair flow. Pair it with a rock tee and moto jacket. A good floppy toque will look so cute on you, too. Just like your shoes, you're drawn to belts with some hardware, like studs or rivets. When it comes to jewellery, you like to go bold with larger scale chains, a studded bangle, and ear cuffs all the way up your pretty ears!

Preppy/Classic

Baseball caps are the ultimate preppy hat. Not only are they functional because they keep the sun out of your face, but, let's be honest, they also can grant you one more day before you have to wash your hair! A few preppy classics I think are good to have are the New York Yankees baseball cap in black and the LA Dodgers in blue. A white Panama hat will look great in the summer. You like plain or braided leather belts in neutrals like black, brown, or tan. You love a headband and probably look best in simple silk or velvet. When it comes to jewellery, you love the classics—no surprise!—such as a strand of pearls, a tennis necklace, and a simple watch.

Sporty

If you are sporty, this is your domain. There are lots of very cool hats made from technical fabric that will work for your style and let you work out in them. I love a good golf visor or a plain black Lululemon or Nike baseball cap. A thick stretchy headband adds life to your ponytail and is perfect paired with leggings. When it comes to watches, there are many excellent digital options in black or bright pops of colour. Count your steps or call someone—you have it all right there on your wrist.

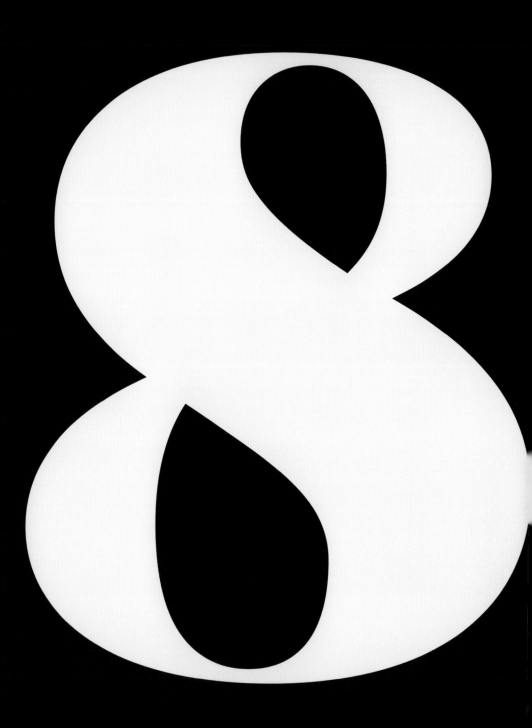

How to Shop

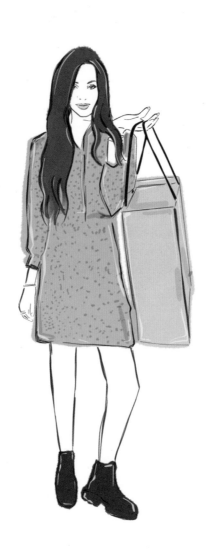

Now that you understand what *your* essentials are (see chapters 1 and 5 for a refresher), you're going to start seeing where the holes in your wardrobe are. Don't feel pressured to go out and fill all those gaps in one shot—in fact, it's better if you don't. What you *are* going to do is make a plan to fill out your wardrobe with thoughtfully chosen pieces that work for your body, your style, and your lifestyle. So let's get started!

Which colours do you feel best in?

BEFORE YOU SHOP

Make a list of the pieces you need and keep it somewhere you can see it often—maybe tape it to the inside of your closet door? Also, think about your colour palette when you're coming up with your shopping list. Which colours do you feel best in? When you wear that chocolate brown sweater, do you get a million compliments? Or do you always feel pulled together when you're in navy? By picking a couple of key shades that will make up the bulk of your wardrobe, your closet won't look like a box of Skittles. And knowing your palette means that, when you're in a store, you'll know to skip colours that look pretty on the rack but don't really belong in your wardrobe. It doesn't mean you can't add a pop of colour here and there—of course you can!—but the bulk of your clothes should be in your palette.

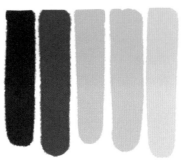

Palette

Get Ready

When you do go shopping now, it's not going to be like the shopping you've done in the past. You're not meandering through stores, grabbing whatever catches your eye. You're on a mission! You are shopping with purpose! You have a list! When I take a client out shopping, I always tell them it's best if they take some time first to feel good. Have a shower, do your hair, put on some lipstick and an outfit you like yourself in (but see the next section). Trying on clothing is less fun when you're not feeling your best. Remember that, even in between trying on new things, you're going to be looking in mirrors all day. And if your hair is a mess and you're wearing an outfit that doesn't flatter you, it can be easy to become discouraged.

What to Wear

Now is not the time to put on a tight-fitting dress, turtleneck, or boots with a million buckles. You want to wear items you can easily slip in and out of. Here are my tips:

→ Wear your favourite bra—it's probably the one you wear most often.

→ Wear underwear with the least VPL (visible panty lines).

→ Wear flats—like loafers or ballerinas—that you can just step into.

→ Wear a loose-fitting dress or a T-shirt with an open neckline so that your face and hair don't get squished every time you pull it off.

→ Bring an old scarf or bandana to use as a "makeup" scarf: put it over your face when you're pulling on a top or dress to protect both your makeup and the garment.

Fuel Up!

And another thing—make sure you eat something before you hit the shops. Nothing is worse than being grouchy the whole time because you're hungry. Remember: you're a snack, so have a snack.

Plus One or No One?

Should you, or should you not, shop with someone else, like a friend or your sister? Do ask a friend whose style you admire, as she's likely to help you find a store's hidden gems. Also, choose a friend who will tell you (nicely!) whether something looks good on you or not. Don't go with a friend who always regales you with the latest gossip—you'll be distracted. Regardless of who you invite, let them know what your goal is for the shopping trip.

WHEN YOU'RE SHOPPING

Find a Knowledgeable Salesperson

Whenever I go into a store, I find someone on the floor who exudes energy and whose style I like, and I ask them what in the store they are loving right now. Of course, I let them know what I'm looking for, but I want to know about what I might not notice myself. They are in the store often, maybe even every day, and they see every piece and how they fit. Now you have an ally—they'll run around and pull all the items you're looking for and then some. It makes shopping so easy! You can also ask them how they suggest the item be styled, and what other pieces in the store would go with it.

Private Shopping

Lots of stores offer a private-shopping service now, and it's usually free. You can call and book a private-shopping appointment, letting the shopper know what you're looking for, and they then go around the store, pulling items in your size and creating looks for you. The clothes will be ready and waiting when you arrive for your appointment. It's fabulous! This is a really fun way to accomplish the task, and many of these private shoppers don't put pressure on you to buy. This is not their first rodeo, and they are looking to build a relationship with you that lasts more than one shop. So, enjoy the champagne and the relaxed environment and have a lovely time.

Hire a Personal Stylist

You know what you need, your closet is clean and ready—this is the best time to hire a personal stylist. The advantage of hiring an independent stylist is that they work with multiple stores, not just one department store. They can help you pick out the best pieces at each. They aren't affiliated with any one department store, and they don't make money off anything you buy, so you won't feel any pressure whatsoever. To find a personal stylist, ask from recommendations from well-dressed friends, staff at boutiques, or even an agency that represents stylists in your area, then google search the names you've gathered and check out their websites. Also take a look at their IGs. If you love the way they dress, they may be the right person for you to work with.

Splurge or Save?

Where to splurge and where to save? It's the million-dollar question. I always suggest to my clients that they splurge on the basics. There's a good chance that a good-quality moto jacket, blazer, or classic nude pumps will last for well over 10 years, so spending some money on them makes sense. If you divide the cost of an essential piece by the amount of times that you have worn it, the cost per wear will be really low. When it comes to your it-list essentials, buy the best you can afford. It's better to have one good-quality purse than a dozen cheap but poorly made ones. You will have that good-quality purse for a long time, and ideally you'll feel confident every time you use it.

The question I get asked most often is "Where can I save a bit?" My answer: save on the really trendy items—pieces that really may not make it to another season. So if you want a pair of trendy sequined booties, that should be where you save. Find these trendier items at a budget-friendly store (like Zara or H&M), or even at a consignment shop.

Buy or Leave It

When you find a potential item, think about how it will work with your existing wardrobe. Does it cross an item off of your essentials shopping list? Does it go with at least three other pieces? Does it suit your body and your style? If it meets these three requirements, then it is worth it! If you're on the fence, or find yourself coming up with elaborate scenarios the piece might work in, take a break. Put the piece back on the rack and go get a coffee or lunch. Give that fashion fever a chance to settle down before you revisit the garment. And if, on second look, it doesn't meet the requirements listed above, leave it at the store.

Mistakes We All Make

Having given you the rules for great shopping, I must confess that mistakes happen even to the most experienced shoppers. There are a few common mistakes that I see clients (and sometimes even me) make. Look out for these traps:

* *Sizing*: Don't get caught up on the size of a garment. Each brand is different. You could be an XS (extra small) in a fast-fashion brand but just squeeze into an L (large) in a European label. Make sure the clothing fits properly, the size on the tag be damned! Buying a garment in the size you want to be rather than what fits just means you'll never wear it. There is nothing worse than muffin tops and tight armpit holes because you bought something in the wrong size. I get it: when you have to size up—or down—to fit into something, it can feel like a personal failure. But it is not. There is such a disparity in sizing between brands that the number on a label basically means nothing. Nobody knows what size you're wearing—they only notice you looking fabulous in that dress or sweater. And, if it really bothers you, cut the tag off.

* *Random mall wandering*: I like a mindless wander-through shops as much as the next person. It's fun to just see what's out there. But for our purposes, we're shopping to complete our perfect, personalized wardrobe. So, think about the items you need and where the best place is to get them. Head straight there and stay focused. You can buy the random lip balm and the plug for your phone later.

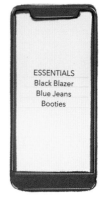

ESSENTIALS
Black Blazer
Blue Jeans
Booties

* *Shopping on vacation*: It's fun to bring home a holiday souvenir—but make it something small and inexpensive. Go for the colourful sarong if you're in the Caribbean, even if you know it won't go into high rotation. Do

not splash out on an Irish tweed suit that doesn't even suit your style.

→ *Blowing the budget:* It's true that shopping causes a dopamine release—we have all been there. You walk into a store looking for a white T-shirt but get caught up in all the other gorgeous items . . . and suddenly you're walking out with bags and bags of stuff you don't need. Of course, it's not the end of the world to veer off your list, but if you spend all your money on non-it-list items, you're going to be as frustrated as ever. And broke. Put your list in your phone and keep circling back to it, just like you do when you're at the grocery store, otherwise you'll end up potentially buying a ton of stuff you don't need.

POST-SHOPPING

Alterations

I know I've been telling you to buy only clothes that fit, but there *are* a few exceptions. Something that is almost perfect can be made completely perfect with an alteration. A high-end boutique will be able to recommend a tailor they trust. And many dry cleaners also offer tailoring services. The most common alteration is for length—in trousers, a dress, or a skirt. This is a quick and inexpensive fix. Another frequent alteration is for sleeve length of a jacket or coat. Anything more complicated than that—like taking a waist in or out—is less of a sure thing. A good tailor will be honest with you about what is and isn't possible. Whatever the garment is, be sure to bring along to the tailor the other items you'll be wearing with it that will affect fit. So, for trousers, bring the shoes you'll pair them with; for a winter coat, bring a sweater rather than a T-shirt for underneath.

Looking after Your Clothes

Clothes will last a lot longer if you care for them properly than if you don't. Read the care instructions on the sewn-in tag and follow them. Even if the tag says you can put the item in the dryer, I remain suspicious of dryers. The heat is what will shrink garments and basically beat-up fabrics. If you've got space, hang-dry shirts and dresses, and roll sweaters up in clean towels to squeeze out excess moisture, then lay them flat to dry. If hang-drying your laundry is impractical, just be sure to keep them in the dryer for the shortest time possible. Silks and fine knits can benefit from special detergents, such as Eucalan or Laundress. For truly delicate or fragile items, handwashing is the way to go. Both Soakwash and Eucalan are mild and don't even need to be rinsed out, making the job much easier.

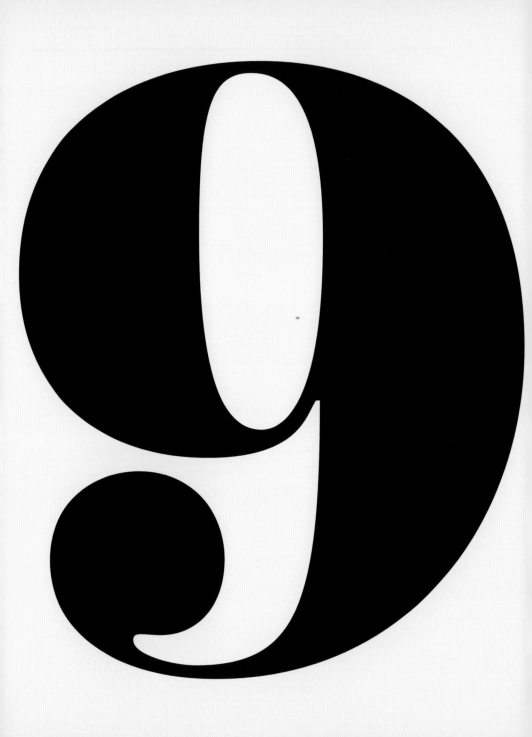

How to Actually Get Dressed

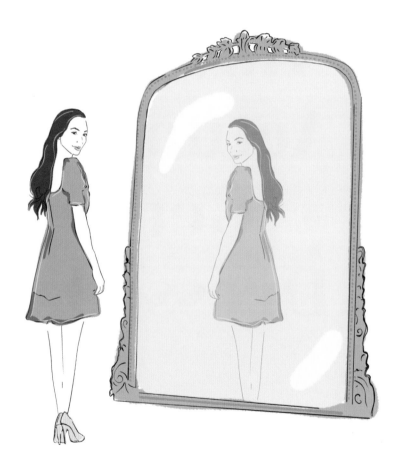

We've cleared, cleaned, and shopped, and now it's show time! There is an important step we still need to take—let's create some outfits. You may feel like doing this before you actually need to get dressed is a waste of time, but believe me, giving this some thought ahead of time will save you time in the long run. Having a few "never fail" outfits on hand and in mind is so important, because if you are short on time, you can get out of the house quickly and still feel pulled together. I suggest having three looks ready and hanging together at one end of the closet so they are visible.

PLAN AMAZING OUTFITS

But how do you put together these outfits?

1. Think about all the situations you're likely to be in. Everyone's life is different, but usually the broad categories are work, going out, and running around. Consider what those scenarios are in your life. Do you need an outfit to make you feel powerful in a meeting? Do you need a dress to wear to a wedding or other big event? Do you need a look you can run errands in but also wear to meet up with girlfriends for a glass of wine?

2. Start with one of your essentials that, by now, you know suits your body and your style. Let's say it's a pair of trousers. Try them on with a few different tops, like a crisp shirt, a slouchy sweater, or a silky tank. Now add a belt and shoes, and maybe a bracelet. Play around until you have an outfit that you know will work in your life.

3. Take a selfie. Or have a friend or family member take a picture of you. It doesn't have to be a glamour shot—it's just to help you remember outfits.

4. Don't stop at the selfie! See what else you can match with those essential trousers. How does a turtleneck switch things up? What about a blazer? By playing around this way, you may find that the trousers you thought were for work only become right for going out for dinner, too.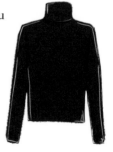

5. It's also worth taking some time trying on garments in unexpected combinations. For example, take your favourite work suit and break it up: try the trousers with a sweater and sneakers, and pull the jacket on over a dress. Or wear a sweater over a dress—now the dress looks like a skirt. Tie your dress shirt in a knot and wear it with jeans. Wear a shirt unbuttoned over a T-shirt or cami as a jacket.

6. If you have a piece of clothing or shoes that you love but can't figure out how to wear—and I hear about this scenario all the time from clients—I have the answer. (And it may sound familiar, from chapter 7.) Search a description of the item in Google Images, along with the phrase "street style." So, for example, "red heels street style," "long green cardigan street style," or "chunky Chelsea boots street style"—you get the idea! You will get pictures of people wearing a similar item and all the ways they have styled it. Use that as a starting point and build from there.

7. Keep creating outfits for all the major activities in your life, always starting with an essential. Ultimately, you want a few outfits for everything you do, from work to getting groceries.

Because I've gone through this process myself, I've learned that one of my favourite dresses—a long-sleeve, leopard-print silk midi—can look professional with chunky loafers and an oversized blazer, it can be dressed up with heeled boots and a trench, or get casual with funky black sneakers and a moto jacket. If I hadn't played around in my closet, I wouldn't know how versatile the dress is.

Tip: Plan for all temperatures. There is nothing worse, in my opinion, than arriving at a venue and feeling too cold or too hot. The key is to dress in layers so that you have options.

GREAT OUTFITS YOU CAN'T PLAN FOR

Of course, one can't anticipate every situation in advance. So, what do I do when I have to get dressed for a scenario I didn't plan for? I always start by considering the venue and the "audience." Is it a cozy, old Italian restaurant with friends, a brunch at someone's house, or a work event? From there, I pick the one item that represents the general vibe of that scenario and build it out from there.

→ If it's a nice restaurant with wood walls, cozy chairs, and dim lighting, I tend to dress in darker colours and mix up the textures; perhaps I'll go a little old school and wear a wool sweater, blazer, and headband.

→ If I'm heading to a modern art gallery that has stark white with bright pops of colour, I might pick up my colour game as well and have fun with it!

→ If I'm attending a conference for work, I'll err on the side of formal. I never know who I might meet there, and I'll want to make a professional impression. Whatever your industry's dress code, be on the buttoned-up end of it. You can always add personality to an outfit of a crisp white shirt tucked into tailored trousers with jewellery or a colourful belt.

What If You Don't Know What the Plan Is?

I suspect we have all, one time or another, been invited to a dinner, work gathering, or some other event and not been sure what the dress code was. If you dress up too much, you feel overdone; not enough and you feel a bit schleppy. The best way to tackle this clothing dilemma is to dress slightly nicer than what you think the general dress code is. However, the key to feeling great is to keep it understated. I had a client who panicked when new friends invited her to an informal dinner at a restaurant she didn't know. She put on a silk leopard skirt (good choice; it hung nicely and was a midi length) and added a white collared shirt (also a good choice). Then it went slightly wrong when she reached for her gold sparkly mules and large hoop earrings. When she arrived she saw that it was a quaint Italian restaurant and that her friends were dressed casually. She would have nailed it, even in heels and a skirt, if everything else have been toned down—she would have been just perfectly overdressed.

MIXING DRESSY WITH CASUAL

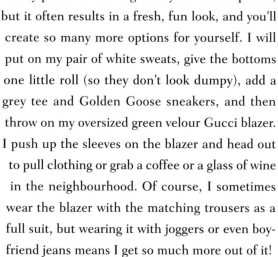

To extend the life of your wardrobe pieces, mix dressy and casual pieces together. Don't be afraid! It may seem counterintuitive to mix a dressy piece of clothing with your casual pieces, but it often results in a fresh, fun look, and you'll create so many more options for yourself. I will put on my pair of white sweats, give the bottoms one little roll (so they don't look dumpy), add a grey tee and Golden Goose sneakers, and then throw on my oversized green velour Gucci blazer. I push up the sleeves on the blazer and head out to pull clothing or grab a coffee or a glass of wine in the neighbourhood. Of course, I sometimes wear the blazer with the matching trousers as a full suit, but wearing it with joggers or even boyfriend jeans means I get so much more out of it!

FOUR BASIC LOOKS YOU CAN RELY ON

After all this, I feel like this chapter wouldn't be complete without my sharing with you a few good looks that can be adapted for almost every body type. Keep in mind that you will tweak these according to your own style and the season.

1. **Classic White Button-Down + Jeans:** Use your imagination and your newfound knowledge of your body type to work with this template. It could be an oversized button-down with a pair of navy skinny jeans, your shoe depending on the season— loafers for spring and fall, white sneakers in spring or summer, boots in winter. It could be a fitted button-down with wide-leg jeans and heels. It could be an open button-down with a white tank underneath and ripped jeans. It's a basic, go-to, no-fail outfit. You 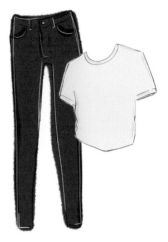 can wear it to coffee, brunch, a meeting, even to the park with your kids (as long as you don't mind if it gets dirty!).

2. **Black Dress:** Depending on the season and your style, this is an easy, classic piece that you can dress up or down. With a longer cotton dress in the summer, you can throw on slides and add a tote or a jean jacket if it's cooler. A long-sleeve knit dress works well in the fall and winter—add combat boots or riding boots for a quick look. Top it off with a blazer or coat if it's cooler outside.

3. **Black Leggings + Oversized Blazer (or Cardigan):** I'm talking about the dressy leggings you have in your closet, whether they're knitted, leather, or patent pleather . . . you get the idea. These can be worn dressed up with a silk tank, oversized blazer, and booties for an everyday look. Sub out the boots for heels in the evening. You could also add cute white sneakers, a relaxed

tee, and an oversized long cardigan for a weekend casual vibe. The leggings will serve you well; they can take you from the school pickup to dinner quickly and are comfortable.

4. **Boyfriend Jeans + White T-shirt + Coat:** Relaxed jeans and a white tee are always a standard uniform to have ready to go. Topping this look with a peacoat, a trench, or a moto jacket will all give you slightly different looks.

I hope I have given you the tools to create your own ideal wardrobe, and that you have enjoyed the process. Remember it's not *just* what you are wearing that makes an outfit appear effortless and stylish. It's knowing what looks good on *you* and what suits your beautiful body shape—ultimately, feeling comfortable in what you are wearing. We also can't forget the most important part, which is that your inner energy and happy soul will elevate any outfit you put on. When you exude confidence and charisma, beauty and style will happen on their own.

The world is ready for you. Now get out there and share your gifts looking and feeling great!

When you exude confidence and charisma, beauty and style will happen on their own.

Style
Charts

Although I've gone into detail about which items of clothing, footwear, purses, and accessories you'll want to make up your own essential wardrobe throughout the book, I thought it would be useful to have a reference you can turn to, to see what may be missing in your closet. I've organized these charts by body type, so go to the chart that that matches your body type, then find your style, and you'll see the essential jacket, top, bottom, dress, footwear, and bag for you. And if you're not sure which body type or style type you are, then go back to the beginning of the book, please!

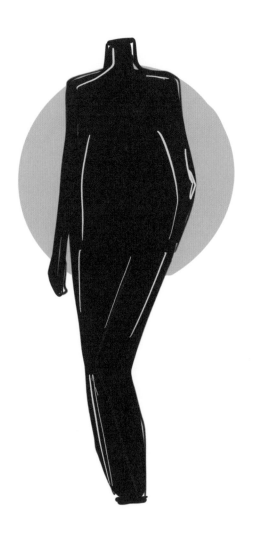

Circle

Known fondly as an "apple," your waist is the widest part of your body, while your shoulders and hips are narrower or about the same width. Although you may or may not have a big bust, for balance, your best bet is to create the illusion of a smaller waist. You want to highlight your best parts, usually your legs or bust. Bright colours are fabulous on your lower body, details on dress hemlines draw the eye to your legs, and tops with diagonal lines, big prints, and texture are great for you. Purses that work for you are structured boxy bags with short handles. Avoid bags that cross your mid-section, as they will add volume there. Chunky shoes with colour and detail will draw the eye downward.

Circle

	Jacket	Pant	Top
Boho	Straight cardigan	Flowing linen	V-neck blouses
Casual	Long open sweater	Wide-leg jeans	V-neck tee or open-neck blouses
Edgy/ Grunge	Fitted leather	Side-fastening straight-leg pleather	Round-neck, wide sleeve
Preppy/ Classic	Structured blazer	Flat-front wide-leg trousers	V-neck collared shirt
Sporty	Straight windbreaker	Flare leggings	Deep V-neck tanks

Dress	Footwear	Purse
Ruffle-hemmed	Wedge shoes or boots	Structured tote
T-shirt dress with empire waistline	Calf-length boot	Top handle bag
Black silk midi wrap	Studded boots	Bowling bag
Knee-length shift	Ballet flats	Rectangular tote
Cotton tank dress	Round-toe sock sneaker	Short handle bag

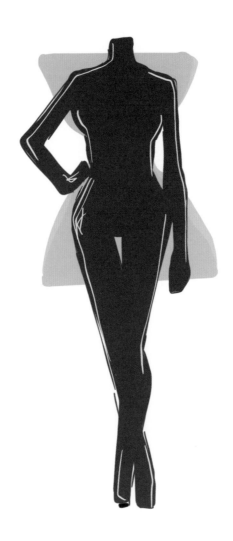

Hourglass

Hourglass bodies have hip and chest measurements that are nearly equal in size, and a smaller waist. Your body is naturally balanced, and the key to dressing for you is to highlight your body's natural shape. You want to choose clothing that shows off your silhouette and keeps it relatively uncluttered. Necklines for tops are any shape that is open, off shoulder, square, scoop, or V-neck; fitted sleeves are perfect for you. It's best if your tops nip in at the waist; stay away from anything boxy. Since you have a balanced silhouette, choose pants that fit at the waist—you want to avoid adding material at your smallest point. Keep your pants on the slimmer side and stay away from pleats, darts, and embellishments. Choose dresses that draw focus to the waist—wrap dresses are fabulous on you.

Hourglass

	Jacket	Pant	Top
Boho	Short jean jacket	Wide leg	Peplum
Casual	Belted cardigan	Bootcut	Fitted wrap
Edgy/ Grunge	Fitted leather moto	Straight cut	Fitted tee
Preppy/ Classic	Fitted blazer	Slim cut	Fitted shirt
Sporty	Crop bomber	Leggings	Fitted tee

Dress	Footwear	Purse
Peplum	Wedge sandals or cowboy boots	Cross-body
Shift	Golden Goose sneakers	Waist-length shoulder bag
Panelled waist	Pointy booties	Leather cross-body
Wrap	Pointy stilettos	Clutch
Bias cut	Sneakers	Nylon bum bag

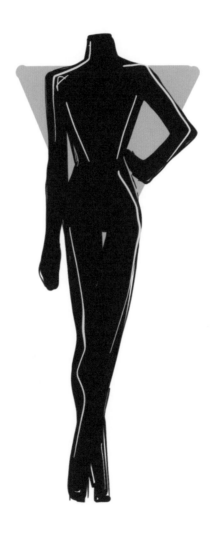

Inverted Triangle

Your shoulders are broad, your hips are narrower. The goal for you is to balance the broad top half of your body with the smaller bottom half. You want to add curves to the hips and bottom and attempt to create a defined waist. Tops that work well for you are deep Vs or those with a scoop neckline that breaks up the shoulder and chest—also shirts that flare from the waist, wrap tops, and darker solid colours. Jackets that give a waist are perfect for you—look for belted ones, and jackets that flare or have deconstructed, fluid lines. Pants that work well are any that add volume, so flares, wide leg, palazzo, and flowing fabric. If you want to wear fitted pants, straight or a cigarette style will work best. Dresses that work well are those that add volume to the bottom half, like a shift dress or A-line dress. Choose shoes that draw the eye down and add "weight"—think chunky and fun! Purses that work for you are those with long straps and that sit on your hips, and also belt bags.

Inverted Triangle

	Jacket	*Pant*	*Top*
Boho	Deconstructed velvet or linen blazer	Wide leg or flares	Deep V-neck tee, tank, or sweater
Casual	Long chunky knit sweater	Straight-leg jeans or boyfriend cut	Jean shirt
Edgy/ Grunge	Moto, belted at the waist	Cigarette crop	Deep V-neck tank
Preppy/ Classic	Blazer with peplum waist	Wide leg trousers or jeans	Turtleneck or button-down shirt
Sporty	Long windbreaker	High-waisted joggers	Deep V-neck workout tank

Dress	Footwear	Purse
Flowing long A-line	Lug-sole army boots or Birkenstocks	Cross-body textured purse
A-line	Platforms	Hip bag
Black silk, empire waistline, or bias cut	Lug-sole Chelsea boots	Cross-body, crinkle leather
Full, pleated	Chunky loafers	Classic tote
Tennis	Chunky sneakers	Belt bag

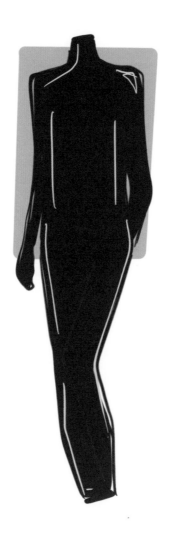

Rectangle

Your body shape has equal bust, waist, and hip measurements. Although rectangles tend to be long and lean, there are size 2 rectangles and size 12 rectangles. Even if not all rectangles are the same, the same principles apply. Your best bet is to define your waist with a belt, to create softness up top. Look for round necklines or V, scoop, or sweetheart. Choose sleeves that have some volume and add interest; avoid tight, shapeless sleeves that will make you look linear. Have fun with bold and or patterned fabrics; thicker fabrics that have some movement will give you the best silhouette. When it comes to jackets and other outerwear, look for garments that are belted or nipped in at the waist. For purses, clutches that are tucked under the arm or slouchy hobo bags work—anything that's soft and adds curves.

Rectangle

	Jacket	*Pant*	*Top*
Boho	Duster coat	Flowy linen flares	Ruffle-sleeve tee
Casual	Wrap coat	Wide-leg jeans	Scoop neck
Edgy/ Grunge	Moto	Leather crop flares	V-neck
Preppy/ Classic	Trench	Wide leg with movement	V-neck tee or sweater
Sporty	Straight cut, mid-length	Cargo	Round neck, long sleeve

Dress	*Footwear*	*Purse*
Empire-line	Clog	Slouchy hobo
Wrap	Ugg boots	Soft bucket bag or tote
X-line	Oval-toe boot	Soft pouch
Shift	Tennis shoe or loafer	Baguette style
Athletic, with cinched waist	Round-toe sneakers	Cross-body belt bag

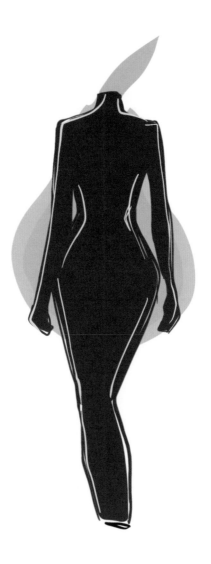

Triangle

Your pear body shape is characterized by hips that are wider than your bust and shoulders. The pear shape is heavier on the bottom, so your goal to create balance is to draw attention upward to your waist and upper body. Focus on pieces with bright colours, texture, and prints on top, as well as structured shoulders. Fitted pieces that accentuate your waist are fabulous. Keep pieces on the bottom uncluttered and clean, and watch out for skinny and tight bottoms, which can emphasize your hips. Keep your necklines wide, and keep volume at your shoulders. Pointed shoes elongate legs, and chunky heels and wedges work well, giving you height and stretching the leg. Choose purses that fall between your waist and hips.

Triangle

	Jacket	Pant	Top
Boho	Long kimono in a dark, slimming colour	Dark-denim flares or wide jeans	Off-shoulder or ruffle-sleeve tee
Casual	Cropped denim	High-rise bootcut jeans	Horizontal-striped tee
Edgy/ Grunge	Cropped moto	High-rise bootcut	Basic black that hits at the waist; pockets on the bust
Preppy/ Classic	Long blazer with shoulder pads	Black straight-leg	Puff-sleeve blouse
Sporty	Cropped bomber	High-rise flare leggings	Bright-coloured tee

Dress	Footwear	Purse
A-line	Pointy suede ankle boots or cowboy boots	Mid-sized embellished-strap colourful shoulder bag
Wrap	Flatform Ugg boots or platform sandals	Mid-sized tote
Empire-line	Tall moto boots	Cross-body bag
A-line	Black or nude pointy pump	Mid-sized tote
Fitted-waist flare	Black or white sneakers that give some height	Bum-pack worn across the body

ACKNOWLEDGMENTS

I would like to thank my parents, Heather and Harold Westdal. Thank you for giving me the best start in life, sharing your values, love for travel, spirit of adventure, and for the educational experience that really set my life into motion. You have always stood behind me cheering me on. And Dad, all those books you made me read, I think they paid off! I love and appreciate you both.

To my sweetest family, my husband Greg and our three outstanding children Aspen, Ryder, and Grayden, I am beyond grateful to be blessed with you all. Thank you for believing in me and supporting me (and for attending all the fashion shows, shoots, and events!). I always wanted to show you my world and it's been so fun to have you there from the beginning.

To my little sister Kristin, thank you for being my first muse, my first "baby", and so loyal and protective of your big sister. You have such a confident, solid energy and I love you to the moon. I feel grateful to have a sister that I can also call a friend.

To my dear friends, old and new (you all know who you are!). Thank you for your support, guidance, and your encouragement. It's been quite the fashion journey. Honourable mention to Erin Hicks for being my first fashion assistant and being there for all the crazy moments and Toby for your voice of reason. Tamara M. for listening to me talk about the "charts" for hours on end, and Nicki for your positive encouragement during the final writing phase of this book.

To my freelance copyeditor Ceri Marsh, thank you for working so diligently and taking my (sometimes disorganized) manuscript and shaping my words into something flowing and fun.

To my illustrator Nessa, thank you for the beautiful illustrations, and the many conversations along the way that made me laugh.

To my publishing team, Rachel Brown and Robert McCullough, thank you for believing in me, this project, taking it into the world, and providing it a wonderful home.

To my clients and followers, you have been my source of inspiration and greatest teachers over the years. It has been a privilege to serve you and I thank you all.

And lastly, if you want to connect with me in person, want to hear me talk more about what I've covered in this book, or just want inspiration, please head over to my YouTube channel. I am blessed with the most amazing community of "XO" friends there, and we would love to have you join us!

INDEX

A

accessories
  belts, 98
  hair, 97
  hats, 97
  jewellery, 91–96
  scarves, 98
  by style, 99–101
alterations, 114–15

B

belts, 98
body type
  bags for, 81–83
  circle, 12, 15, 55–56, 133–35
  determining, 12–15
  essentials for, 55–57
  footwear for, 66–67
  hourglass, 12, 15, 56, 137–39

inverted triangle, 12, 15, 141–43
and measurements, 17
rectangle, 12, 16, 57, 145–47
triangle, 12, 16, 57, 149–51
boho
  accessories, 99
  circle shape wardrobe suggestions,
    134–35
  essentials for, 58–59
  footwear for, 68, 135, 139, 143,
    147, 151
  hourglass wardrobe suggestions,
    138–39
  inverted triangle wardrobe
    suggestions, 142–43
  purses/bags for, 83, 135, 139,
    143, 147, 151
  rectangle wardrobe suggestions,
    146–47

style type, 20
triangle wardrobe suggestions,
    150–51
boots. *See* footwear

C

casual
    accessories, 99
    circle wardrobe suggestions,
        134–35
    essentials for, 58
    footwear for, 68, 135, 139, 143,
        147, 151
    hourglass wardrobe suggestions,
        138–39
    inverted triangle wardrobe
        suggestions, 142–43
    purses/bags for, 83, 135, 139,
        143, 147, 151
    rectangle wardrobe suggestions,
        146–47
    style type, 21
    triangle wardrobe suggestions,
        150–51
circle body shape
    boho style, 134–35
    casual style, 134–35
    described, 15
    edgy/grungy style, 134–35
    essentials for, 55–56
    footwear for, 66, 133, 135
    preppy/classic style, 134–35
    purses/bags for, 82, 133, 135
    sporty style, 134–35
    wardrobe chart by style, 133–35
closet
    cleaning of, 29–34
    organizing, 43–47

uses of, 27–28
clothing. *See also* essentials
    alterations to, 114–15
    caring for, 115
    and closet cleaning, 30–38
    creating outfits, 120–22
    donating used, 32, 36–37
    folding, 46
    four basic looks, 124–26
    grouping in closet, 45
    hanging, 46
    mixing styles, 124
    recycling used, 32
    selling used, 37–38
    suggestions by body shape and
        style, 133–51
    for unplanned situations,
        122–23
clutches, 80–81, 139, 145
cross-body bags, 79–80, 139, 143,
    145, 151

E

edgy/grunge
    accessories, 99–100
    circle shape wardrobe sugges-
        tions, 134–35
    essentials for, 59–60
    footwear for, 68–69, 135, 139,
        143, 147, 151
    hourglass wardrobe suggestions,
        138–39
    inverted triangle wardrobe sug-
        gestions, 142–43
    purses/bags for, 84, 135, 139,
        143, 147, 151
    rectangle wardrobe suggestions,
        146–47

style type, 21
triangle wardrobe suggestions,
    150–51
environment, fashion industry
    impact on, 35
essentials
    by body type, 55–57
    boho style, 58–59
    bottoms, 54
    casual style, 59
    for circle body shape, 55–56
    cocktail dresses, 54
    day dresses, 54
    edgy/grunge style, 59–60
    for hourglass body shape, 56
    for inverted triangle body shape,
        56–57
    jumpsuits, 54
    preppy/classic style, 60–61
    putting together, 55
    for rectangle body shape, 57
    sporty style, 61
    by style type, 58–61
    tops, 53
    for triangle body shape, 57

F
footwear
    basic wardrobe, 65–66
    for boho style, 135, 139, 143,
        147, 151
    caring for, 72–73
    for casual style, 135, 139, 143,
        147, 151
    for circle body shape, 133, 135
    for edgy/grungy style, 135, 139,
        143, 147, 151
    for hourglass body shape, 139

    for inverted triangle body shape,
        141, 143
    for preppy/classic style, 135,
        139, 143, 147, 151
    for rectangle body shape, 147
    shopping for, 71–72
    for sporty style, 135, 139, 143,
        147, 151
    for triangle body shape, 149,
        151

H
handbags, dressy, 80. *See also*
    purses
hangers, 44
hats, 97
hourglass body shape
    boho style, 138–39
    casual style, 138–39
    described, 15
    edgy/grunge style, 138–39
    essentials for, 56
    footwear for, 66, 139
    preppy/classic style, 138–39
    purses/bags for, 82, 139
    sporty style, 138–39
    wardrobe chart by style,
        137–39

I
inverted triangle body shape
    boho style, 142–43
    casual style, 142–43
    described, 15
    edgy/grunge style, 142–43
    essentials for, 56
    footwear for, 67, 141, 143
    preppy/classic style, 142–43

purses/bags for, 82, 141, 143
sporty style, 142–43
wardrobe chart by style, 141–43

J

jewellery
  bracelets, 91, 93–94
  costume, 95–96
  diamonds, 91–92
  earrings, 91, 92, 95
  gold, 94–95
  metals, 92–94
  necklaces, 91, 93, 94, 95
  pearls, 95

L

lifestyle, 22–23

M

matching concept, 70
measurements
  and body shape, 17
  and brand sizes, 13
  how to take, 13–14

N

neck, length of, 14

P

preppy/classic
  accessories, 100
  circle shape wardrobe sugges-
    tions, 134–35
  essentials for, 60–61
  footwear for, 69, 133, 135
  hourglass shape wardrobe sug-
    gestions, 138–39

inverted triangle wardrobe
  suggestions, 142–43
purses/bags for, 84
rectangle wardrobe suggestions,
  146–47
style type, 21–22
triangle wardrobe suggestions,
  150–51
proportions, 15
purses
  for boho style, 135, 139, 143,
    147, 151
  for casual style, 135, 139, 143,
    147, 151
  for circle shape, 133, 135
  for edgy/grunge style, 135, 139,
    143, 147, 151
  essential, 78–81
  for hourglass shape, 139
  for inverted triangle shape,
    141, 143
  for preppy/classic style, 135,
    139, 143, 147, 151
  for rectangle shape, 145, 147
  for sporty style, 135, 139, 143,
    147, 151
  for triangle shape, 149, 151

R

rectangle body shape
  boho style, 146–47
  casual style, 146–47
  described, 16
  edgy/grunge style, 146–47
  essentials for, 57
  footwear for, 67, 147
  preppy/classic style, 146–47

purses/bags for, 82–83, 145, 147

sporty style, 146–47

wardrobe chart by style, 145–47

S

scarves, 98

shoes. *See* footwear

shopping

decision making, 112

economic aspect of, 111–12

mistakes in, 112–14

with personal stylist, 111

preparation for, 107–9

private, 110

and salespeople, 110

shoulder slope, 14

sizes

and body measurements, 13

and body type, 16

sporty style

accessories, 100–101

circle wardrobe suggestions, 134–35

essentials for, 61

footwear for, 69

hourglass wardrobe suggestions, 138–39

inverted triangle wardrobe suggestions, 142–43

purses, 147, 151

purses/bags for, 84, 135, 139, 143

rectangle wardrobe suggestions, 146–47

style type, 22

triangle wardrobe suggestions, 150–51

style types

boho, 20, 134–35, 138–39, 142–43, 146–47, 150–51

casual, 134–35, 138–39, 142–43, 146–47, 150–51

edgy/grunge, 134–35, 138–39, 142–43, 146–47, 150–51

preppy/classic, 134–35, 138–39, 142–43, 146–47, 150–51

sporty, 134–35, 138–39, 142–43, 146–47, 150–51

sustainability, 35

T

tote bags, 78–79. *See also* purses

triangle body shape

boho style, 150–51

casual style, 150–51

described, 16

edgy/grunge style, 150–51

essentials for, 57

footwear for, 67

preppy/classic style, 150–51

purses/bags for, 83

sporty style, 150–51

wardrobe chart by style, 149–51

W

wardrobe. *See* clothing

watches, 96